**Praise for**

# Alzheimer's from the Inside Out

"Extraordinary, brilliantly insightful, inspirational, courageous, thought-provoking—there is no end to the positive descriptors that can be attached to this amazing book by Richard Taylor. *Alzheimer's from the Inside Out* is not only a *must read* for persons with Alzheimer's and their personal and professional care partners, it is, plain and simple, a *must read* book. In sharing his reflections on, as Richard puts it so uniquely, 'living with Dr. Alzheimer between my ears,' Richard prods the reader to reflect on universally vital questions about values and life in general and to laugh with him about human foibles. No matter how experienced and informed one is about Alzheimer's disease, Richard's capacity to eloquently share his questions and insights causes the reader to stop and re-think and to do it yet again on the second or third reading."

—**Carol Bowlby Sifton,** family caregiver, clinical dementia consultant, editor of *Alzheimer's Care Quarterly,* and author of *Navigating the Alzheimer's Journey*

"After reading this book I have come to the conclusion that this is perhaps the most important book in the field of dementia care ever written. These poignant essays come from the heart and the soul of a sensitive and intellectually gifted man who has become a national champion and advocate for the millions of people living with this disease."

—**Linda L. Buettner, Ph.D., CTRS, FGSA,** Professor of Health Science, Florida Gulf Coast University

"Among the millions with this cruel disease, Richard is rare in that his preserved memory, language, and thinking skills made possible these essays about his experience of the disease. He offers valuable insights to family and professional caregivers seeking to uphold the dignity of all people living with the disease. A debt of gratitude is owed to him, his wife, and his family for refusing to go gentle into that good night."

—**Daniel Kuhn, M.S.W.,** author of *Alzheimer's Early Stages*

"We have treatments, theories, support groups, and resources, but until you read this book, do you really know what it is like to have Alzheimer's? Richard provides a realistic, candid journey through the heart, soul, eyes, and ever-changing mind of one who is living with this disease…we get to walk in Richard's shoes, if only through his writing….It is my feeling that medical professionals, paraprofessionals, family members, caregivers, and, yes, patients would benefit from reading this book to at least attempt to understand the journey that is Alzheimer's, from the inside out."

—**Mischele Warner, M.H.S.,** family caregiver

"By dissecting his own thinking process and the behavior of those around him, Richard Taylor, Ph.D., gives us incomparable insights for appreciating the truths and troubles of Alzheimer's disease. He records in warm, honest detail the organic battle to maintain his personal identity and shares his thoughtful prescriptions for caring, communicating, and advocating in *Alzheimer's from the Inside Out.*"

—**William "Bud" Hunnel,** family caregiver and Former Board President, Alzheimer's Association, Houston and Southeast Texas Chapter

"Written with sensitivity, humor, and passion, *Alzheimer's from the Inside Out* describes the author's sometimes bumpy, but always insightful, journey with Alzheimer's disease. Telling his stories in a series of informative vignettes, Richard challenges us all to be more authentic and work to make life better for persons with dementia—not tomorrow, but today!"

—**Virginia Bell, M.S.W.,** co-author of *The Best Friends Approach to Alzheimer's Care*

"I thought I understood what life was like for my Alzheimer's-affected parents—until Richard's story enlightened me with insight into an unimaginable world. Every family with an elderly loved one, and every medical professional who works with elders, should read this gripping and marvelous book!"

—**Jacqueline Marcell,** author of *Elder Rage* and host of *Coping With Caregiving* radio program

"Practical tips, philosophical musings, and a call to action! This book highlights the challenges in coming to terms with one's *identity* following a diagnosis of Alzheimer's disease and is a reminder to doctors and caregivers alike of the importance of open and honest communication."

—**Helen Regan, M.A.,** Alzheimer's Disease International, United Kingdom

"Dr. Taylor's journey into the fearful horizon of Alzheimer's disease reminds us that no matter what our affliction, we remain human to the end. His story is one of exquisite sensitivity to the sometimes excruciating twists and turns of living with a chronic illness that slowly, progressively, robs him of his sense of self. Rather than the long litany of symptoms and signs to be managed in the biomedical narrative of the disease, Richard Taylor, like Cary Henderson and Thomas DeBaggio before him, confronts us with the experienced reality of Alzheimer's. This is an exceptional book, one that people diagnosed with AD and other dementias should read because they will see that they are not alone, that they are indeed comprehensible. For the rest of us, *Alzheimer's from the Inside Out* is a reminder that we care for *people,* not diseases, and as such, each person's story must be told and listened to."

—**Robert E. Reichlin, Ph.D.,** licensed clinical psychologist and geropsychologist, private practice and voluntary faculty, Department of Medicine–Geriatrics, Baylor College of Medicine

"Richard Taylor's advanced training in psychology as well as his many years as a counselor make him especially able to comment on the relationship changes that have accompanied his worsening dementia. Some people with dementia are unaware of the changes they go through, but not Taylor. He offers his own personal insight into the losses of dementia, and his book is a valuable contribution to the small collection of books authored by people with dementia as they experience their own decline."

—**Charles Schneider,** international Alzheimer's advocate and author of *Don't Bury Me*

"[Richard Taylor] has written a book about how dementia affects not only those who have the disease, but loved ones who stand by to witness the progression of this debilitating disease. Richard is so articulate that caregivers, family members, and medical professionals can now understand what a person with dementia is experiencing because of his first-hand account. His story will help everyone who reads the book gain more compassion and patience."

—**Debbie Ricker, OTR/L,** Executive Director, The Memory Center of Orange County, California

# Alzheimer's
## from the
## Inside Out

# Alzheimer's from the Inside Out

by

Richard Taylor, Ph.D.

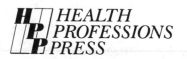

HEALTH
PROFESSIONS
PRESS

Baltimore • London • Sydney

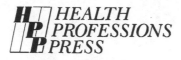

**Health Professions Press, Inc.**
Post Office Box 10624
Baltimore, Maryland 21285-0624

www.healthpropress.com

Typeset by Integrated Publishing Solutions, Grand Rapids, Michigan.
Manufactured in the United States of America by
The Maple-Vail Book Manufacturing Group, York, Pennsylvania.

The opinions expressed by the author are his alone and do not reflect the opinion of the publisher or any other party. None of the information provided in this book is in no way meant to substitute for a medical practitioner's advice or expert opinion. Readers should consult a medical professional if they are interested in more information about Alzheimer's disease, dementia, or related disorders. This book is sold without warranties of any kind, express or implied, and the publisher and authors disclaim any liability, loss, or damage caused by the contents of this book.

The essays on the following pages originally appeared in *Alzheimer's Care Quarterly* (2005–2006, Vols. 6:2, 6:3, 6:4, and 7:1): pp. 3–5, 13–27, 33–50, 54–56, 75–112, 117–118, 148–162, 169–180, 194–195.

Cover photograph © 2006 Kat Pokora, Silverthorne, Colorado.

**Library of Congress Cataloging-in-Publication Data**

Taylor, Richard, 1943–
   Alzheimer's from the inside out / by Richard Taylor.
      p.    cm.
   ISBN-13: 978-1-932529-23-4 (pbk.)
   ISBN-10: 1-932529-23-3 (pbk.)
   1. Mental health.   2. Alzheimer's disease—Patients—Biography.
   I. Title.
   RC523.T39   2007
   362.196′8310092–dc22   [B]                    2006026087

British Library Cataloguing in Publication data are available from the British Library.

# Contents

**II   From the Inside Out**

**III   From the Outside In**

# Alphabetical Contents

# About the Author

This book is a collection of essays written in the five years since Richard Taylor was diagnosed with "dementia, probably of the Alzheimer's type." He lives in Cypress, Texas, with his spouse Linda, and his Bouvier des Flandres (dog), Annie. His son and family live across the street from him. He now spends his days playing with his two grandchildren, gardening, and writing. Originally, he started to write to better understand for himself what was going on inside of him. He writes for five or six hours every day. Even as the disease progresses, he thus far has maintained his ability to look at and attempt to understand himself.

Richard is a passionate advocate for several issues concerning the involvement of people living with a diagnosis of one of the diseases of dementia. He remains an active member of the Dementia Advisory Committee of the U.S. Alzheimer's Association, looking at how to better integrate individuals living with the diagnosis in the leadership, program development, and delivery functions of the Association and its local chapters. He continues to be a sought-after speaker at various professional conferences. He is constantly looking for new audiences, especially of professionals who work in the field of dementia, to help them with getting to know the people they serve.

Richard is an articulate, thoughtful, and thought-filled speaker to caregivers. Hundreds of them have used his insights as the basis for conversations and insights into what might be going through their loved one's minds. Many Alzheimer's chat rooms, across the United States and worldwide, were created in large or small part with his support. He publishes his own newsletter of, by, and for people with dementia.

As this book goes to press in winter of 2006, control of his concentration is sometimes elusive. His language facility is still mostly intact, although he increasingly searches for the right word. His granddaughter Christina is learning to read and to read to him. His garden becomes smaller and smaller each year; he plays bridge (with a cheat sheet) once a week and is halfway through editing another book of his writings.

Richard is always open to exchanging ideas and observations with others. Contact him at *richardtaylorphd@gmail.com*.

# *Preface—The Right Write Stuff*

When writing became fashionable in ancient Greece, Plato complained that writing would end the practice of memorization of poetry and of his own works by the citizens of Greece. Within 30 years, his prediction was confirmed by reality. Most all Greek citizens who previously could memorize hundreds and hundreds of lines of poetry had lost this ability.

He also worried that if people began to write things down rather than speak about them, the writer's ideas might very well be misunderstood by the reader, as opposed to speaking, where the speaker could correct any misunderstandings by the listener on the spot.

Although I am not of Greek heritage, I share Plato's concerns: only my fear is not with the form and content of written documents, it is with dementia, probably of the Alzheimer's type.

I had a mind much like that of an ancient Greek. What I read and heard, I then absorbed like a damp sponge. I was a facts and news junkie. I knew a little about lots, and lots about a little. I didn't have a photographic memory, but I was able to integrate what I read and heard into a fairly impressive body of knowledge in my mind (at least my three-year-old granddaughter and I thought so). I read and thought about anything and everything. I wrestled with the concept of a universe with no edges and I knew three recipes for how to make play dough. I could recall my row and seat number when I was in first grade (row eight, seat seven), and all the bones of the hand. (A friend of mine in medical school once bet me she could memorize all of them before me—she won, but I finally did learn them all. Unfortunately, I wasn't the one in medical school! Thankfully, I have finally forgotten them.)

Today, like the ancient Greeks, I am unable to recall what I once knew. I can't remember new information as readily as I did in the past. Unlike the ancient Greeks I am increasingly finding that speaking as a means of communication is fraught with problems that were not there for me in my pre-Alzheimer's days. I can no longer trust myself to say what I mean and mean what I say, and I cannot recall as accurately my own words as I did in the past.

What to do?

One theory of why writing was invented is that when a shaman invented some dance or chant that preceded something good happening to the people, both the shaman and the people wanted to make sure they didn't forget it. They began to scratch pictures on the walls of caves to remind them what they had done to cause it to rain, or make the pain in the Chief's big toe go away, or make the 6 million locusts all fly away at the same time.

It still makes sense to write things down. If I meet someone I want to meet again, I ask for their cell phone number and write it down on my hand. If I need to repair my car, I look at the scratchings on the yellow pages for the name and number of someone who specializes in the make of my car.

When I figure something out and don't want to depend on my memory, I write it down. As Dr. Alzheimer and his gang of sticky-footed ne'er-do-wells began to tromp around my brain, I quickly lost the ability to easily memorize and/or absorb information I heard and read. As he began to take up residence in my hippocampus and my executive function became problematical, people, even my own family, started to misunderstand me. Since I wasn't too accurate in recalling exactly what I had said, I became less and less able to explain myself to them and—more importantly—to myself. The advantages of speaking as opposed to writing were becoming fewer and fewer.

Increasingly, I couldn't understand myself and other people couldn't understand me. What was happening? Why was it happening? What did it mean?

Of course the medical professionals were of little or no help to me. They still don't know what causes this disease, how and why it progresses, and the 10 million dollar question: how to cure it. Enter Mr. Google. He didn't have any answers either, but he sure knows a lot about it and he was willing to sit with me until I had asked and he had tried to answer all of my questions. He was able to write out his answers and give me as many copies of them as I wanted, so that later on, at my leisure, I could reexamine them. He went all over the world trying to help me. He found people who were dealing with the disease, researchers, and health care professionals who had dedicated their lives to helping people in my exact circumstances. What a find!

Now, what to do with all this information, much of which I was forgetting almost as fast as I was reading it, and even when I remembered it I wasn't confident I was understanding it completely. I sat down in front of my computer and started to take notes. When I had created a few summaries on the same subject I would read them and think about them and try to find insights into myself and my experiences.

As thoughts are wont to do, they would pop up unannounced—at night, for example, just before I went to bed. By dawn's early light I would discover that I had forgotten all of it completely.

I tried a version of my own shorthand to recall insights into myself. I either couldn't read them because my handwriting had deteriorated to the point where even I couldn't read it, or the short-handedness of the words made no sense to me other than during the moment at which I wrote them down.

I tried carrying around a small tape recorder to capture my thoughts for future examination. I felt uncomfortably like Donald Trump: "Note to self, do something about your hair." I lost—or, as I chose to characterize it, *misplaced*—several tape recorders. I was so uncomfortable pulling a tape recorder out of my pocket and talking to myself OUT LOUD, I gave up on the idea.

I always came back to writing them down. "Them" consisted of worries I had about the future, insights I had into my own behavior, questions for which I had no answers, and observations I had about myself and my caregivers. Over time, the observations became broader and deeper. I started to amuse myself and to affirm that I still had some creative abilities yet working. I began to weave and wrap my thoughts into short essays, sometimes based on a quotation by someone else and sometimes based on my own thoughts. I found out that if I could save enough thoughts and organize them by theme—read them one after the other—I could weave an essay that was sometimes interesting, sometimes funny. Most of these essays were short, no more than a couple of pages in length.

Writing became my "therapy without a co-pay." It was a way for me to attempt to figure things out for myself, or at least think about them and recall what I had concluded. I seldom solve a problem about which I am writing, but I feel more confident in myself because I can reread my thoughts. There is less a sense of "what's the use" when I try to figure out what is happening to me, what will happen to me, and why things are now happening to me. It is, no doubt, my way of trying to maintain my sense of control over what is going on between my ears—by understanding what is happening to me, to my brain, to my thought processes, and to my relations with others.

One day I was discussing with a friend an issue common to most individuals living with early Alzheimer's disease. I asked him if he would read one of my essays and share his reactions with me (he too was living with early Alzheimer's). To my complete surprise, he really liked what I had to say and how I had said it. He showed it to his care-givers and they actually made copies of it to share with other distant family members.

I shared some of my writings with my local Alzheimer's Association, and they asked if they could print one of my essays in their newsletter. Since then, my essays have appeared on their web site, on the web sites of dozens of groups, and in a number of professional journals. Many people have asked my permission to show my work to their families and friends, and teachers in the field have shared it with students. I am honestly flattered and still surprised.

I don't write for others: I write for myself. I write to better understand myself, to remember my own insights, to work through my own issues, to find the right questions to ask, and to find a few answers to give myself. I write to entertain myself and reassure myself that some of the old me is still here.

Thanks to technology—Google, grammar checkers, spellcheckers, on-line dictionaries, and fascinating web sites on most anything anyone can imagine—I appear to be close to who I was before Dr. Alzheimer's extended visit between my ears. Friends read my writing and say, "Oh, you don't have Alzheimer's disease." I respond: "Because I can still think? Because, when given a day, I can produce two pages of writing that used to take me 10 minutes?"

I would encourage people with a disease that alters their thinking to *write;* not just a journal of what happened today or a dozen to-do lists for tomorrow. Think about yourself, your caregivers, your relationships, your present, and your future—and *write.* Think about what you wrote, and write again. Just the process of writing can be reassuring. Writing about things can be immensely helpful when talking about them is no longer working. Write lots, and write every day. Scratch down ideas, and then go write. Show your writing to others. Talk about it with your caregivers. Show it to fellow travelers on your road seldom taken, and encourage *them* to write. It worked and is working for me. It has morphed from a hobby into a part of my daily routine. I miss it on the days I don't find time to write. Writing has become a confirmation to me, of me, and by me. Some people believe "they think, therefore they are." I write, therefore I am.

—*R. T.*

# A Note from Linda Taylor

I have been married to Richard for more than 20 years. He was a remarkable human being when I first fell in love with him, and I believe with all my heart he still is. Now he is remarkable in new ways. Since he first started to write this book after being diagnosed with Alzheimer's disease, I have been a helpless and troubled witness to the deterioration of his cognitive abilities.

For the past 5 years, Richard's annual neuropsychological tests have tracked his very slow but steady decline. Perhaps it is only in my mind, but I see him maintaining some plateau of ability and then over the course of a month falling off the plateau to a lower level of ability. He sits for hours and hours in front of his computer, writing and rewriting until he is satisfied with what he has written. What previously took Richard 10 minutes to write now sometimes takes 10 hours. Occasionally, he swears at the computer and at himself because he has just erased or misplaced something he spent hours working on. Everyone has a solution to offer him; fewer and fewer solutions seem to work for him. His computer is in constant need of repair. He tries to make it work and to fix it by himself, and then our son comes over once a month to undo his tinkering.

Early on, Richard discovered a voice recognition software program that allows him to speak while the computer types for him. You would be painfully aware of his deficits if he typed a letter without this assistance, because now he can seldom see his own errors on the screen. Thank heavens for spell checkers and grammar checkers—as long as he remembers to use them. He gets so upset with himself when he discovers errors in his e-mails long after he has sent them to someone, but most of the time the mistakes are invisible to his eyes and his brain.

Richard becomes confused easily now, especially in a new environment. I cannot leave his side in an airport, for example, because he becomes disoriented and may wander away. Although he continues to advocate for the rights of people with Alzheimer's and to travel to conferences, he can no longer go by himself. It is too much of a risk for Richard, and for me. I worry about him when he is away. A family member or friend always accompanies him to speaking engagements. He cannot drive, does not like to read, and has trouble concentrating to complete a task. When he paid the same bill three times in 1 week, emptying our checking account, we decided it was time for me to take over the family finances.

Richard has become very restless. He searches for words. Whereas before he had too many things to say, he now says too little, especially in the evenings. If more than one person is talking, he can't understand what either one is saying. Recently I have observed that when he is not in control of a conversation, and he is unable to change the subject in order to be in control, he is quite liable to lose the thread of the conversation. Sometimes, he responds in conversations about two sentences late.

Perhaps most unsettling to Richard is the fact that he now sometimes "misses" what is going on around him. He just cannot seem to understand some things and some time frames. It frustrates us both. Also unsettling to me is the fact that his personality is changing. He is more withdrawn into himself. He is more defensive in our discussions/arguments. He says he understands what I am saying, but he does not.

One of his doctors told me that intelligent people are better able to conceal the impact of Alzheimer's disease. I thank God that Richard was born very intelligent. Even now, to speak with him (except late in the evening), most people wonder if he really has Alzheimer's disease. I know. I know for sure. I denied it to myself in the beginning. For several years I held out hope that something else was changing my husband. There is no doubt in my mind . . . although I find myself sometimes still hoping.

It is strange how others imagine that someone with Alzheimer's disease should act and how they should think. I am pretty much resigned to the fact that I will never understand my husband as I did before this horrible disease entered his life. I hate this disease!

Watching him mow our lawn is one of my saddest sights. Richard has lovingly tended our lawn and his gardens for many years. He is so proud of "his" lawn, but you can almost see the changing patterns in his mind revealed by the path of the lawn mower. He seldom finishes the job. He becomes distracted and starts doing something else before he's finished cutting the grass, and he has not a clue that this has happened.

I wish you knew Richard before Alzheimer's disease changed his life and my life. I am so glad you will at least have the chance to get to know him as he was several years ago through the essays that are collected in this book. I have learned things about him and about us by reading his essays. I do not always agree with him, but he always has been and still is a remarkable person.

Welcome to Richard's early years of thinking about and living with Alzheimer's disease. I believe there are insights here for everyone—people living with Alzheimer's disease, their caregivers, and those as yet unaffected by a disease of dementia—who seek a clearer and better understanding of the issues that Richard, and others like him, now confronts every minute of his life.

I will continue to love this remarkable man forever.

*Linda Taylor*
*November 2006*

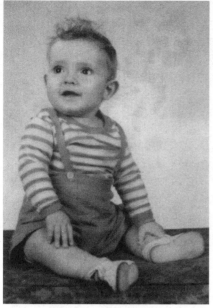

The early years

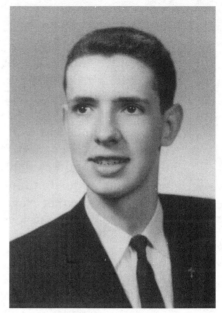

High school graduation

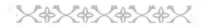

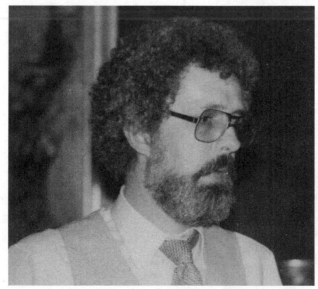

The hippie period

*Richard Taylor*

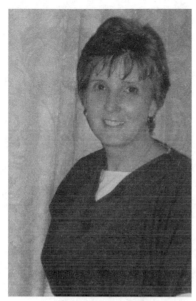

Linda—
*My Champion or My Hero?*
(p. 163)

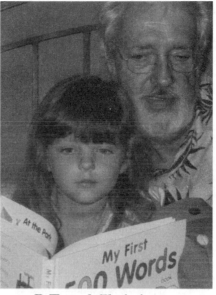

R.T. and Christina—
*"I Can Read." "I Can't"*
(p. 97) and *Christina, Mrs.
Hippopotomus, and Me* (p. 154)

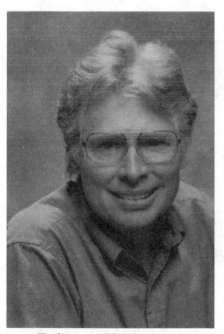

Robert—*Hemingway,
Alzheimer, and Taylor* (p. 62)

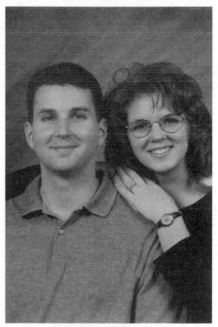

Jason and Shannon
*There Is Something (More)
Wrong with Dad*
(p. 204)

# What Is It
# Like to Have
# Alzheimer's Disease?

Alzheimer's (*AHLZ-high-merz*) disease is a progressive brain disorder that gradually destroys a person's memory and ability to learn, reason, make judgments, communicate, and carry out daily activities. As Alzheimer's progresses, individuals may also experience changes in personality and behavior, such as anxiety, suspiciousness, or agitation, as well as delusions or hallucinations.

The disease is the most common cause of dementia. Dementia is a collective name for progressive degenerative brain syndromes that affect memory, thinking, behavior, and emotion. Symptoms may include:

- Loss of memory
- Difficulty in finding the right words or understanding what people are saying
- Difficulty in performing previously routine tasks
- Personality and mood changes

Dementia is not a normal part of aging. It knows no social, economic, ethnic, or geographical boundaries. Although each person will experience dementia in his or her own way, eventually those affected are unable to care for themselves and need help with all aspects of daily life. There is currently no cure, but treatments, advice, and support are available.

*http://www.alz.co.uk/alzheimers*

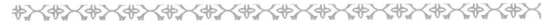

# Jesus, Albert, Alzheimer's, and Richard

XΦXΦXΦXΦX

*Intelligent people understand others.*
*Enlightened people understand themselves.*
—Lao Tzu

After spending years fruitlessly searching for a historical record of a person named Jesus, Albert Schweitzer concluded that when someone told him about Jesus they were telling him more about themselves than Jesus; so, too, with Alzheimer's and these essays. There is little historical record of and by individuals living with Alzheimer's disease. First-hand accounts of the disease are few, and all end about the same time in the progression of the disease: Stage 3—when the disease forever blocks the individual's ability to provide self-reports of the disease's impact. On the other hand, there is a growing body of personal journals by caregivers of people with Alzheimer's.

Like the Gospels of the New Testament, these recollections attempt to recapture the essence of a loved one through a collection of the loved one's words and actions. Like the Gospels, they are more the reflections and perceptions of the writers than the loved one. When placed next to each other, they do not always agree. They sometimes contradict each other. They do not all include the same words and events. Since there is no record of what the loved one actually said and thought, readers are left with their own interpretations of the second-hand recollections. So, too, with Alzheimer's disease. No one who has the disease has ever returned from her or his demise and presented "the truth" of Alzheimer's. As the disease engulfs a mind, the ability to report what is going on within the mind is lost to the outside world. This is my attempt to leave a record of what is going on between my ears. I am writing

> *This is my attempt to leave a record of what is going on between my ears. It's not the medical record. It's not the personal account of my life. It's not a psycho-social report.*

about the disease as it is expressed by and is having an impact on my mind, my perceptions, and my world—as I perceive the process. I make no claims to speak to "the Alzheimer's experience." Although I have spoken to hundreds of individuals in early-stage, many in second-stage, and a few in late-stage Alzheimer's, no one sees the disease, him- or herself, or caregivers exactly as do I. There is no one Alzheimer's experience which, if understood, becomes the key to understanding individuals with the disease.

However, there do seem to be some concerns and reactions that can be generalized to many individuals with the disease. It is to those general concerns and experiences I hope these essays speak. I speak of them as I have experienced them.

There is no doubt that my own "issues," life experiences, and perceptions flavor these essays. But, I have tried not to bore you with "this is your life, Richard," and instead present you with "this is how I am living my life as I share my brain with Alzheimer's disease."

When I started to write these essays, it was not my intent to address them to caregivers. I wrote to clarify for myself what was going on with and in me. Then, I showed them to a few other people who shared my diagnosis of early-onset, early-stage Alzheimer's disease. I saw their eyes brighten and sometimes fill with tears as they read of some of their own experiences in my writings. It was then that I decided to share my writings with others. I wanted others to know they are not alone with an Alzheimer's changing mind. There are others with them on the Alzheimer's road less traveled who are uneasy about the present and the future, and unable to figure things out as they have in the past. It is in my nature to think about thinking. I have never been shy when it came to speaking. Some folks don't think much about their thinking processes. Some don't think (or worry) about the future. Even fewer think about how thinking and the disruption of our thinking processes affects our future. I do.

When I have shown these writings to many caregivers, they have asked me pointed questions from their perspective. How do I think they could best engage me or others with the disease in ways that would be supportive and more in tune with their loved ones' inner thoughts and needs?

I do not want to become an advice columnist on caregiving. I do want caregivers to read my writings and figure out for themselves how this information and these insights can help them understand, appreciate, and honor their loved ones. Finally, to readers who do not have the disease and are not responsible for anyone with the disease but realize the bell could toll for thee: This is a record of my thoughts and my life, and it may not exactly "fit" your life. I hope the fears, issues, and problems that Alzheimer's disease has raised in my life will encourage you to think about your own life in ways you may not have considered previously.

When people tell me about their Alzheimer's experiences, I, as with Schweitzer and his conversations with people about Jesus, know they are telling me more about themselves than about "the Alzheimer's experience." We have no proof of the Alzheimer's experience. In fact, no one really knows if the people who have been told they have "dementia, probably of the Alzheimer's type" really have Alzheimer's disease. The fact will not be established until they die, and then only if they had previously given permission for their brain to be removed and examined for the medical signature of the disease.

# There Is No Such Thing as Alzheimer's Disease!

The hour, the day, and most of the month after my neurologist said to me, "You have dementia, probably of the Alzheimer's type," my spouse, my family, my friends, and certainly I, worried, cried, and ran as fast as we could down the first hundred steps of the spiral stairway to depression. The assemblage of doctors who followed me for more than a year met with me on almost a weekly basis. They stuck me, jabbed me in my spinal cord, and removed what seemed like gallons of my blood for analysis in labs located from Houston, Texas, to Princeton, New Jersey. They asked me, by actual count, 102,000 questions about everything, from "Did you or do you lick walls painted with lead paint?" (no, to this question) to "Can you recall who was the 17th president of the United States?" (Andrew Johnson). One year and one month after I first went to my GP and told him my daughter had mentioned to my wife, "There is something wrong with Dad," I finally got a less-than-definitive diagnosis—13 unlucky months later.

Dementia is a pattern of symptoms indicative of some disease or combination of diseases. It is, I read, both progressive and degenerative. It affects individuals' thinking, behavior, memory, emotions, and personality.

Alzheimer's disease is the most common cause of dementia. Memory loss, especially short-term memory loss, is the most common early symptom, later leading to disorientation as to time and place, inability to solve the everyday problems of life, and changes in personality and abrupt changes in mood.

Neurologically and certainly psychologically, diseases that attack the brain are especially threatening to human beings because they inevitably lead to a time when we will be, but not be, ourselves. Prior to that point in time, we will be aware of the process but increasingly be unable to do much about it. Welcome to my world.

From a psychopharmacological perspective, drugs may or may not temporarily delay the progress of the disease, but they make no claims to stop or cure it. New medications currently in the pipeline make similar claims, but all concede that shortly after the drugs lose their effectiveness there will be little difference between those who took the drugs and those who did not. The average life span of individuals living with the diagnosis is 10 years from the date of the diagnosis. Again, welcome to my life span and my world.

Another way of looking at it: Alzheimer's disease, on average, subtracts 10 years from the expected life span of an individual. That is probably my future.

How dare I claim there is no such thing as Alzheimer's disease, especially when I am someone living with the diagnosis? One reason is that I knew the title would attract attention. Another reason is that no one seems to know for sure if anyone who is currently alive actually and for certain has the disease; this, of course, includes me. The doctor says you have dementia, "probably" of the Alzheimer's type. Only after you die and they pop open your head and inspect your deceased brain can they say for sure, sort of, if you had it. (Of course, at that point you're dead and probably won't care.) Currently, approximately 4 million people in the United States are living with a diagnosis of "dementia, probably of the Alzheimer's type." Is this claim for any one individual based on the evidence produced by the autopsies of the previous 4 million people who lived under this doctor-made cloud? Of course not! Is this after-the-fact verification the best way to make a diagnosis? Of course not, especially a diagnosis that is associated with such a profound impact on caregivers and on the diagnosed individual.

> *How dare I claim there is no such thing as Alzheimer's disease, especially when I am someone living with the diagnosis?*

"We have identified a number of symptoms which, when they occur together, we can probably label the owner of these symptoms as having dementia, probably of the Alzheimer's type," claim the contemporary neurologists. My response is that "probably" is neither definitive nor reassuring that your diagnosis is accurate. It would be, if I believed this bundle of symptoms is unique to the disease and exclusive of other diseases. But, of course, it isn't. There are lots of other diseases with symptoms that include memory loss, dysfunctional executive activity, misperception of spatial relationships, and so forth.

The multiple symptoms that identify each of the syndromes of the diseases of dementia are not, in fact, mutually exclusive. They may not even capture all of the syndromes that are broadly labeled as *dementia*. We now know there are more than 20 kinds of cancer, yet we still call 20 different disease processes *cancer*. We now know that senile dementia is not a single room full of specific symptoms. Right now, we claim it is a large house full of different rooms, each of which uses the address of "Dementia Drive," but each room claims its own apartment name: Alzheimer's, Lewy bodies, vascular ischemic stroke, etc.

Now why, you may be asking yourself, should this be of any interest to someone living with the diagnosis of "dementia, probably of the Alzheimer's type"? The diagnosis of Alzheimer's disease is still primarily based on first identifying the symptoms and checking to see that they meet the agreed-on syndrome labeled *Alzheimer's disease*. Second, tests are given to check that these symptoms are not due to any known cause. If the symptoms are there, to the levels measured by self-fulfilling tests, and we can't identify what causes them, then physicians pronounce, with lowered eyes and a restrained voice: "You have dementia, probably of the Alzheimer's type." Many of them, I have noticed, forget the *probably* part and imply certainty!

Under the collective breath of medical society, they sometimes whisper as we are leaving the room, dissolving in our own tears: "Of course, we still don't understand the exact process in your brain which is producing these symptoms. In fact, we still don't understand the exact processes of a healthy brain which is not producing these symptoms. We have yet to all agree on where, why, and how we remember, or forget. Lots of us have guesses based on our specialties, personal interests in research, availability of subjects, what kind of imaging hardware is available to us, and how much the reputation of our institutions helps us in securing funding." Ask three respected researchers in the field of Alzheimer's disease "What causes the disease?" and you are sure of getting at least two different answers and at least one "I don't know."

So, physicians know almost for sure that I have Alzheimer's disease because I exhibit a certain group of symptoms that were long ago labeled as evidence of a disease named after Dr. Alzheimer. And besides, they can't find any other cause of the symptoms. And the few times they are able to examine the remains of the few people who permit such examination, they find the same gross anatomy in the examined brains. And when they see the same types of brains post-mortem which Dr. Alzheimer saw, they label the disease *Alzheimer's disease.* Of course, they aren't sure that other diseases or conditions might cause the same or similar results in dead people's brains—Alzheimer's disease is currently their best guess.

My good friends the neurophysiologists have made it easy for us to decide whether or not we have Alzheimer's disease. Score very, very near on the end of a continuum of scores on a memory test, and score in the same relative position on another test measuring one of four other constructs, and you have Alzheimer's disease. (Of course the neurophysiologists dare not make a medical diagnosis; that, through powerful lobbying efforts, still remains the exclusive property of physicians.) It sure sounds persuasive doesn't it? Six hours of testing, lots of graphs, numbers, and statistics so complicated to accurately derive that computers are used to calculate them; and they all suggest one conclusion: *dementia, probably of the Alzheimer's type.*

In fact, we don't know if symptoms progress equally or evenly on a predictable time schedule. We don't know if the measurable symptoms progress predictably between individuals. We don't know within a day or a month when someone moves from Stage 1 to Stage 2, and we can't agree on how many stages there are to the disease. What we do claim to know and measure is based primarily on the observation of caregivers and professionals. Subjective as these observations are, they do not easily form a firm foundation upon which to base statistical analysis.

Therefore, psychologists know (but can't tell me directly, because that might be construed as a diagnosis) that I probably have Alzheimer's disease because of the answers I gave to a total of about 1,000 questions from a battery of tests. When they compare my answers and scores on these tests (composed of my sex, age, family history, current medications, mental health history, ethnicity, gene types, eye color, height, and shoe size—you pick what you believe are the active variables because they don't have any proof, just guesses) with those of a preselected group of people, my results match the results of people who already have been diagnosed as having Alzheimer's disease. No, in most cases this is not true. My scores match people who have been labeled as having the same *symptoms* as me. Wait, this is getting confusing. Exactly my point. The more it is explained, the more it is clear that there is uncertainty; the probability of the results being accurate predictors of something which is at best "fuzzy" is questionable, especially given that these results are supposed to support the grave claim: "You have dementia, probably of the Alzheimer's type."

I am neither a physician, nor a researcher, nor a health care professional who for years has worked in the field of Alzheimer's care and research. I am not a philosopher or an ethicist. I am not a professional writer who looks into WMDs last week, the plight of giraffes in the New Orleans zoo this week, and something about Alzheimer's disease next week. I am, I repeat, someone who heard the words "you have dementia, probably of the Alzheimer's type" directed at him, by a neurologist I admired and trusted.

Perhaps, just perhaps, there is probably no such disease as Alzheimer's disease. Why should you or I care?

You should care because you probably might now be a caregiver or know someone who has been diagnosed as probably having the disease. I have been diagnosed with the disease. Unfortunately, through the years and for reasons not now of primary interest to me, the probability of the diagnosis has been replaced by the inevitable consequences claimed to be caused by the disease: the slow and sometimes caustic erosion of self; the death of the current self; the replacement of the current self by someone who is most times unlike and sometimes at least perceived as the antithesis of the former self; and the deterioration of that self into helplessness and death.

We should care because the mere thought of living the life associated with this disease has a profound impact on many lives. My choice of medications is based on the claim "this treats Alzheimer's disease." My sensitivity to myself and my behaviors is based on "this is what happens to people diagnosed with Alzheimer's disease." My future is clearly defined by "this is what happens to people with Alzheimer's, this is the order in which it happens, and this is how it ends. Watch this video and you can see it happening to other people!" My finances are measured against a different set of expectations. My family and friends see me through different eyes and readjust their behaviors around me accordingly.

A national Alzheimer's association, with over 60 local chapters, has a vision of "a world without Alzheimer's." Every year, millions of people walk to promote research to make this vision a reality. Hundreds of books are written, careers are built, and TV talk show episodes are produced around the words "you have dementia, probably of the Alzheimer's type."

Instances of rediagnosis with some disease other than Alzheimer's are not now infrequent (as people who like to use double negatives are not not inclined to say). When the bundle of symptoms does not worsen over time; when science finds other explanations for the specific symptoms; when physicians admit to a mistake in their diagnosis (honest, it does happen); when individuals seem "cured" of the symptoms by faith, prayer, plants, vitamins, spirits, their own spirit, minerals, hands, aromas, healers, and an increasingly longer list of other "atypical" and "nonmedical" causes, the mistakenly diagnosed individuals somewhat sheepishly pick up the pieces of their lives and try to move back into their "old selves."

When we are not "saved" from the disease by this or that, we live with the disease. I currently live with the disease. Before, I found some comfort in the word *probably* as in "You *probably* have Alzheimer's disease." But there are no grounds for hope because "I probably have Alzheimer's disease." I for sure have dementia and it is probably of the Alzheimer's type. Maybe I don't have "it." The baseline fact is, I have dementia. It may be that instead of Alzheimer's disease, I may have Pick's disease, vascular dementia, or one of the other 90+ identified diseases of dementia. The more I read about the other identified diseases of dementia, the more convinced I am that they are not all mutually exclusive. The more I read about scientific breakthroughs in basic research on Alzheimer's disease, the more I am convinced that lacking a complete, well-documented, and universally accepted map of the mind and how a healthy mind works ensures we cannot yet identify the root cause of the diseases of dementia. If we don't know how something works, how can we fix it? How will we know it is fixed?

> *There is far too much emphasis on the label, the name, and the symptoms generally associated with the disease, and too little emphasis on the individuals who actually* have *the disease.*

We will end up with an AIDS-like approach. Take this pill and that pill, come back in a month, and we will try some more pills. Here is one pill that replaces six pills—try this, until we come up with individualized cocktails that seem to keep the disease under control. What else is happening between your ears, which is not visible through your test answers and blood, no one will know until we know exactly how the healthy brain operates. Of course, there is always the comforting fact that after you die, we might know for sure if your brain looks like the lady's brain that Dr. Alzheimer examined many, many years ago.

"And my point is?" From my perspective as a person living with the diagnosis, there is far too much emphasis on the label, the name, and the symptoms generally associated with the disease, and too little emphasis on the individuals who actually *have* the disease. Researchers are beginning to realize that, as with cancer, there may be no "magic bullet" which in and of itself causes Alzheimer's disease. It might be caused by a cosmic collision of a number of anomalies. The emphasis is now on delaying the process of cognitive deterioration.

There may never be a cure for Alzheimer's the way we think of a broken arm being cured. Alzheimer's disease (whatever we finally decide it really is) may frequently, or perhaps always, be accompanied by some of the other 20+ diseases of dementia. Those of us who have the disease and those who care for us should concentrate on dealing with the unique package of symptoms Dr. Alzheimer has sent us. Praying, hoping, donating, walking, looking, waiting for a cure is like concentrating on trees that may or may not be real and missing the forest that *is* real. If it is or is not a single disease, or if it will ever be cured, should be at the bottom of our priority list of things in which we should invest our energy.

I know more about Alzheimer's than do many physicians who have treated me. So what? What do I really know? Of what value is it to me? Has it, does it, or will it change my life for the better? Nope!

# What Is It Like to Live in Purgatory?

> The First Level of Purgatory: You are in Limbo, *a place of sorrow without torment.* You encounter a seven-walled castle, and within those walls you find rolling fresh meadows illuminated by the light of reason, whereabouts many shades dwell. These are the virtuous pagans, the great philosophers and authors, and others unfit to enter the kingdom of heaven. You share company with Caesar, Homer, Virgil, Socrates, and Aristotle. There is no punishment here, and *the atmosphere is peaceful, yet sad.*
>
> —Summary of Limbo
> (http://www.4degreez.com/misc/dante-inferno-information.html)

My admittedly ignorant understanding of purgatory (I am neither a theologian nor a Catholic) is that reasonably good people who have done some bad things in their lives (isn't that most of us) spend an indeterminate amount of time living between heaven and hell. The living conditions get progressively worse depending on how bad you were and how long you are being retained in purgatory. You have no idea when you will find out if you are going up or down. The decision is not yours to make.

Welcome to my purgatory—the time between knowing I might have Alzheimer's disease to the time I knew for sure I had Alzheimer's disease.

My entire family had not been together since last Christmas. On the way to the airport, my daughter leaned over and whispered into my wife's ear, "There is something wrong with Dad." I had noticed that I was increasingly more forgetful. Nothing out of the ordinary, I thought, just more of it. I felt a little more distant from everyone, but that comes and goes in all of us. I just was not as involved in the world as I used to be. I chalked that up to aging. Could I be a tad short tempered? Moody? Paranoid? Surely not me!

A month later, while at my general practitioner's for my annual checkup, I mentioned my daughter's comment and my own

> *Welcome to my purgatory—the time between knowing I might have Alzheimer's disease to the time I knew for sure I had Alzheimer's disease.*

observations of myself. "Don't worry," he said, "We have a medication for people with Alzheimer's."

"ALZHEIMER'S DISEASE? No way! I'm too young. I take good care of myself. I don't eat meat. I think good thoughts at least once every day. I perform random acts of kindness, sometimes! I am friendly to stray dogs and cats, although I don't actually take them home with me. Mother Teresa, I'm not, but I don't deserve the curse of Alzheimer's disease!"

Off to the neurologist for a year's worth of testing, a year in purgatory. I read books, checked dozens of Internet sites, made frequent trips to my local Alzheimer's Association chapter, and checked out and viewed a dozen depressing videos of individuals in the later stages of the disease.

Living in purgatory was getting worse.

Stick me in my spine (three times!), inject radioactive something into my blood, and scan my brain again and again and again. Was I eating lead paint? Do I cook in aluminum pots? Do I have AIDS? Did I live near a chemical plant and eat the dirt in my backyard? The questions and the tests went on and on. Each time I thought this would immediately lead to the defining moment, and then there was another test. Other than my immediate family, I told no one about where I was living or why I was living there. Each day I dressed for work, left purgatory, and pretended nothing was wrong and nothing was going to be wrong.

Finally, finally, THE day arrived.

"Dr. Taylor (I had asked him to call me Richard), you have dementia, probably of the Alzheimer's type."

What he said after that, no one in my family can remember! Doctors claim the diagnosis is inclusive rather than exclusive, so why did they schedule so many tests that revealed nothing? Why did they exclude causes of something other than Alzheimer's with endless, costly, and occasionally painful tests?

I guess that's just the way life is in purgatory.

Now I realize that purgatory is better than my real-life alternative, to live the rest of my life with Alzheimer's disease.

Nonetheless, there being no choice, since I have yet to "pass on," I have moved out of purgatory and back into the world of the living—but now I must live with and in Alzheimer's disease!

# What Is It Like to
# Have Alzheimer's Disease?

✕✛✕✛✕✛✕✛✕

What is it like to drive your car from Houston to Anchorage? The answer depends on many things: the type of car you will drive, the age of the car, how well you maintained it, where you are in your trip, if others are helping you with the drive, if you have enough gas or access to a gas credit card, if you have accepted the fact you must drive to Anchorage, whether or not you are afraid of arriving in Anchorage.

What is it like to have Alzheimer's?

This, too, depends on many things: Do you have an existing group of individuals who are committed to your well-being? Are you a proactive or a reactive person when it comes to dealing with doctors, your health insurance company, and yourself? Where do you live: Houston, Texas, or Houston, Nigeria? Do you have insurance? Especially long-term care insurance? Does your culture and economic class encourage and promote younger generations taking responsibility and care of their family's older generations? There are dozens of important factors outside of yourself that will directly and significantly influence you and your inner experiences with the disease.

After meeting, speaking, and corresponding with hundreds of people who have Alzheimer's, I am convinced there is no universal answer to the question, "What is it like to have Alzheimer's?"

Since the disease process unpredictably and seemingly randomly destroys various cognitive processes and undermines the basis of most all understanding and memory, each person has a unique and personal way of dealing with the rate, the degree, and the various components of the syndromes we attribute to Alzheimer's disease. Neurologists who tell us they understand the disease because they see 4 or 40, or 400, individuals with Alzheimer's does not mean they understand me or you. Just as there really is no single "average" person, there is no meaningful "average" Alzheimer's disease experience.

I was diagnosed with dementia of the Alzheimer's type *two* years before I wrote this piece. I imagined, maybe hoped, that some day I would wake up and a heavy velvet curtain would have fallen during the night. I would wake up to a world where I could see shapes but not enough details to know what or who they were, sort of like Plato's flickering shadows on the wall produced by the fire on the cave floor.

Instead, right now, I feel as if I am sitting in my grandmother's living room, looking at the world through her lace curtains. From time to time, a gentle wind blows the curtains and changes the patterns through which I see the world. There are large knots in the curtains and I cannot see through them. There is a web of lace connecting the knots to each other, around which I can sometimes see. However, this entire filter keeps shifting unpredictably in the wind. Sometimes I am clear in my vision and my memory, sometimes I am disconnected but aware of memories, and other times I am completely unaware of what lies on the other side of the knots. As the wind blows, it is increasingly frustrating to understand all that is going on around me, because access to the pieces and remembering what they mean keeps flickering on and off, on and off.

Thanks in large part to my family caregivers, I am still functioning in the non-Alzheimer's world. I drive, I learn (although I seem to forget much of what I learn), I teach, I love, I mostly understand—but not all the time, and not always the way others do. It is a constant effort to look around the lacy webs and to have to put effort into understanding and doing things that came naturally but a few months ago (cooking, reading, driving to a new store, remembering the recent past). Some activities hide beyond the knots and rarely have clarity (arithmetic, reading a watch, remembering what I just read). It is not a lot of fun, but I can still do it!

> *Individuals have a cold, have cancer, have the measles. Alzheimer's has the individual.*

Does the disease increasingly dominate my life, or has the disease insidiously and largely unconsciously become a part of my life?

Does the chicken come first, who I am?

Does the egg come first, Alzheimer's disease?

Today, but not yesterday, I firmly believe: Individuals have a cold, have cancer, have the measles. Alzheimer's has the individual. Ask me again tomorrow!

I am trying to be rational and realistic, using tools that are rusting and increasingly out of sync with each other. In my writings you will feel me leaning one way in one paragraph (*I am in a war with this disease and I will go down fighting. This is an opportunity for me to grow in ways few people have an opportunity to experience*), or another way (*I'm mad, I'm sad, and I feel sorry for myself. Why won't others join my self-pity party?*).

My writings don't offer answers, just my own observations from my own increasingly unsure perspective.

# They Are Glad They Caught It Early. Am I?

I have talked with dozens of people in their 30s and 40s who have been diagnosed with early-onset (defined as anyone under 65 who is diagnosed), early-stage (the first of a three-stage description of the disease) Alzheimer's disease. I was 58 when I was officially diagnosed. After hearing the diagnosis, I cried every day for three weeks. My neurologist told me that 95% of the people he diagnoses with Alzheimer's are not even tested. The patients, most of whom are in their mid-to-late 70s, would not be able to understand the instructions, let alone answer the questions in a reliable manner. I was tested for a year, and I understood everything that was going on. I still do. Right now, I just forget a lot.

> *I was 58 when I was officially diagnosed. After hearing the diagnosis, I cried every day for about three weeks.*

I now feel a sense of accomplishment when an hour goes by and I am not made aware of my illness by someone correcting me or asking me a question I cannot answer. However, soon there is old Dr. Alzheimer with his pitcher of ice water to throw in my face. He reminds me it was the illness that caused me not to lock the front door at home, or to leave the dog in the yard for almost a day, or to forget to do this or that. I now almost never stop being aware of the illness. What was an occasional disruptor became a bother and is now a constant companion and reminder of my journey down the road less traveled.

When I was first diagnosed, I joined a support group, and all of the members were older than I. Most of them denied they had the disease because—I believe—they could not conceptualize it. Since they didn't understand it, why should they believe others who told them they had something they couldn't see, feel, or conceptualize? The group leader encouraged us to tell each other how we felt. Most all of them felt okay. They were a little irritated that they could not drive or handle money, but for them life was mostly on track.

For those of us who "caught" it relatively early in life, and in whom it was diagnosed early in the progression of the disease, we know what is going on. We can still entertain meta perspectives on our own behaviors, our minds, or ourselves. We know that we are off life's track. We know we are wandering farther and farther away from the crowd, our families, and ourselves.

Although I am aware of the fact that I have Alzheimer's disease, this awareness doesn't always help me to make the most of my situation, or to ask for or accept the help that I sometimes need.

My neurologist may be happy he made the diagnosis early on in the course of the disease. I am not so sure it was such a blessing.

# WHAT ARE SOME LESS
# COMMON FORMS OF DEMENTIA?

- Pick's disease affects personality, orientation, and behavior. It may be more common in women and occurs at an early age.

- Creutzfeldt-Jakob disease is caused by an infectious organism. Symptoms include memory and behavioral problems and a loss of coordination. The disease progresses rapidly along with mental deterioration and involuntary movements.

- Vascular dementia (multi-infarct dementia) results from a series of small strokes or changes in the brain's blood supply. Blood clots block small blood vessels and destroy brain tissue. The strokes interfere with the function of daily activities and cause memory problems and slurred speech.

- Huntington's disease is an inherited degenerative disease. The disease causes involuntary movement and usually begins during mid-life. Other symptoms include disorientation, personality changes, impaired judgment, and memory and speech problems.

- Parkinson's disease is a progressive disorder of the central nervous system. The symptoms include tremors, speech problems, stiffness of limbs and joints, and physical movements. In later stages of Parkinson's disease, some patients develop dementia.

- Lewy body disease symptoms are similar to those of Alzheimer's disease and include memory problems, confusion, language problems, and difficulty recalling current events. Individuals with Lewy body disease experience hallucinations and can become fearful.

*http://www.helpguide.org/elder/alzheimers_dementias_types.htm*

# The End of Act One.
# And Now, an Intermission
# of Indeterminate Length

*The play's the thing*
*Wherein I'll catch the conscience of the King.*
—William Shakespeare, *Hamlet* (II, ii, 633)

For most of my caregivers, Alzheimer's disease produces a play within a play. I still play the roles of the husband, dad, friend. I also now am playing the part of someone who has a disease that affects my cognitive functions. I have seen Alzheimer's disease described in three stages, five stages, nine stages, and most recently in 12 stages. I have always thought of it as a disease in three acts. The first act is the semiprivate act. The script is mostly within my own head. Only those around me really know I am not "myself" but I am, in effect, acting the part of my old, pre-Alzheimer's self.

After an intermission of indeterminate length, during which I hang around the lobby and slowly deteriorate to the point where I cannot go back on stage and pretend that I have not changed who I was and how I previously acted, the curtain rises on the second act. Act Two takes place in a series of increasingly restrictive residential facilities. Places with names like "Peaceful Gardens" and "Tranquility Place" are the mise-en-scène of Act Two.

Act Three takes place in a nursing home, hospital, and perhaps a hospice. It is the end of my play. As people leave the theater, I hope they remember me as I was before we were all forced by circumstances to watch and "act" in the Alzheimer's disease play within a play. One of the reasons I published this book was to "catch the conscience" of my readers, and of my legislators.

My Act One lasted about three years. Most of that time, while I was on stage I was in disguise and peeking out of an almost-invisible closet. Aside from the other cast members (family and close friends), no one in the audience knew about my Alzheimer's disease. What university advertises a faculty of Ph.D.s with Alzheimer's disease? What student would believe a low grade was due to his or her own performance rather than to the plaque-filled Alzheimer's mind of an instructor?

For two of the three years, I won outstanding teacher awards! The third year I was asked privately if I would graciously withdraw from the competition so someone else could win. (I'm not sure if this is a reflection of my teaching ability or the sad state of classroom teaching in general.) On the last night of my teaching career, I sat in a restaurant with my students as they celebrated the end of the semester, and I privately grieved the end of my life as a teacher. That sweet-and-sour meal was my last taste of 20 years of teaching and consulting. I felt the curtain coming down on my own first act as I left the restaurant.

> *What university advertises a faculty of Ph.D.s with Alzheimer's disease? What student would believe a low grade was due to his or her own performance rather than to the plaque-filled Alzheimer's mind of an instructor?*

I now wander around the lobby (my house) until such time that, despite the best efforts of my caregivers, I become a serious threat to myself and/or to others. At that point, the chimes ring, the lobby lights flash, and the stage lights begin to dim. Act Two will begin!

There really isn't much to do during an intermission. You stand around and talk about the weather while you try to nurse one Bloody Mary to last the entire intermission. You have a vague idea what's going to happen in the next act, but you don't talk about it because it might ruin it for other people who didn't even understand the first act. You know that awareness of the play ends with Act Two, but you will still be the star of Act Three. In fact, many of those sitting around you know the same fact, but it just doesn't seem appropriate to talk about that right now.

So, here I sit, in my office at home, having done all I want to do with my garden, having completed all the home repairs I want to complete for the rest of my life, and spending most of my time now writing disease-driven vignettes. I am no longer challenged in the ways I was when I taught. I cannot measure my ability to think and communicate in the same way I did when I was a teacher. I have already completed one round-trip of visiting all my family members.

I know that some time in the near future, door locks will get changed, windows will be nailed shut, neighbors will be on the look-out for wanderers, knobs will mysteriously disappear from the stove, and the oven will stop working. The TV will work, but that's about all that won't change in the house. Not only will my car keys disappear, so will the car! No more unsupervised time with my granddaughters. Pleasant people I don't know will start showing up and just sit around looking at me. They will keep offering to help, but I won't be able to think of anything they can help me with. I will still see, hear, feel, walk, and talk. I will dress and undress myself. No trouble going to the bathroom. Why will they constantly be hovering around me?

I have no sense of how long I will be able to enjoy my retirement at home with my family. I had once thought these would be the bright-est days of my life. Work long and hard and then enjoy carefree days in our paid-up house, with no bills and a 401k plan that was growing faster than we could spend it.

I had pictured it in my mind . . . really, what difference does it make what I saw or thought? What counts, what has meaning, is what is. And what is is me: full of self-doubts, fearful of tomorrow, and not fully understanding today. Surrounded by loving caregivers who share many of my fears—self-doubts, fear of the future—yet we do not and cannot share the same state of mind.

Stay tuned . . . I will, as long as I can.

# Cogito Ergo Sum

## *I think, therefore I exist.*
—René Descartes

The French philosopher René Descartes, and many people with early-onset, early-stage Alzheimer's disease, ask questions like, "Where do I fit in? How do I come to myself, my identity? How do (and will) I know I exist?" With apologies to all that follows in Descartes's *Discourse on Method,* I too ponder these questions, not as a rationalist philosopher greatly influenced by thinkers from the Age of Enlightenment, but as someone on the cusp of fundamentally altering the ways I think and what I think.

How will I come back to myself? Who will I be? How will I know I exist? How will I fit in?

Truly knowing the truth about people with late-stage Alzheimer's is like claiming to know the form and content of the fourth or fifth dimension. We are limited by our own thinking and language to imagining something we cannot see, hear, feel, touch, or taste. We can take what we know and project it, but we are still within the confines of our own minds. We are stuck with the evolved network and systems of our frontal lobes. We are still slaves to our primitive on/off brain switches.

We talk to people with the same brain but with different wiring. We ask them questions to try to make them understand us. If I think and I am and you are, therefore you must think something like me—only you are a little "off." We test Alzheimer's diseased brains with questions created by non–Alzheimer's diseased brains, and then claim to better understand the foreign brain.

I simply can't imagine who I will be or how I will think once the semi-transparent veil of Alzheimer's turns into the opaque curtain of Alzheimer's.

I have spoken with people behind this curtain. I have listened to them. I still don't have a clue. What will I be thinking if I become violent? What will I be thinking when I can't swallow any more? The living unknown frightens me more than death. I can understand that once I die, life is over; what happens after that I have no access to as long as I am alive. I can see and talk to people who are on the other side of Alzheimer's, and I still don't have a clue as to what is going on.

For me, knowing makes it less frightening, even if I can't control it. Knowing makes it a new experience, rather than an indeterminate sentence to some form of purgatory.

| *A Joke* | *A Riddle* |
|---|---|
| Descartes walks into a bar | Richard walks into a bar. |
| The bartender asks: | The bartender asks: |
| "Do you want a drink?" | "Richard, do you want a drink?" |
| "I think not," says Descartes. | "I think not," says Richard. |
| POOF! He vanishes! | What happens to Richard? |

Why should I even worry about these questions and answers? I won't even be aware of the change! Why don't I frame it as my death? I will still be here but I won't know or care.

I think I'll be thinking, therefore I am!

Maybe!

---

René Descartes was a famous French mathematician, scientist, and philosopher. He was arguably the first major philosopher in the modern era to make a serious effort to defeat skepticism. His views about knowledge and certainty, as well as his views about the relationship between mind and body, have been very influential over the last three centuries.

*http://oregonstate.edu/instruct/phl302/philosophers/descartes.html*

# My Last Six Words

Now, understand that I do not worry or even think about this on a daily basis. I have not practiced saying them, nor do I even know or care what they will be. In all likelihood I won't understand what I'm saying, and the meaning will be entirely in the minds of my caregivers who hear them.

Having said this, a good friend of mine recently told me that in order to qualify for Medicare coverage of hospice care services, you must be interviewed. One of the standards against which you will be measured in that interview is that you may use and speak no more than five different words. If you speak a sixth word, you are automatically disqualified from Medicare coverage of hospice care expenses.

This has led me to muse about what my sixth word will be. The romantic in me says it will be *Linda* (my spouse), or *love*, or *family*, or the name of one of my grandchildren, or perhaps *Peace Now*. The darker side of me says it will be an angry word, maybe a cuss word, perhaps a hateful word, or a word expressing self-pity. It could be a word expressing pain, fear, and frustration. Realistically, I believe it will be some word randomly chosen by a brain long out of touch with reality. The word will have nothing to do with me or my inner or outer worlds. I can play the same game with words 5, 4, 3, 2, and 1.

> *It is amazing to me to ponder the possibility of missing the ultimate unique moment of my life, my death, because I have no words to describe it, or understand it, or appreciate it.*

Most of the individuals I have seen experiencing end-stage Alzheimer's are mute. They had not uttered a word in many months. Some had not spoken for a year or more. There they sit: simply sitting slouched over in a wheelchair, silent in gaze and in sound.

If I don't have words, if I don't have access to words, will I be thinking? How can I know and understand what I'm feeling if I have no words to describe it? It is amazing to me to ponder the possibility of missing the ultimate unique moment of my life, my death, because I have no words to describe it, or understand it, or appreciate it.

Perhaps I should spend more time today and tomorrow and the next day using the words I have in order to understand and appreciate what is going on inside and outside of me. Perhaps I should tell people what I am thinking and how I feel. Words are the triggers to our higher-level feelings of love, astonishment, fear, beauty. Words like *spouse, family,* and *garden, flowers, the Beatles*—these are words that trigger my appreciation and satisfaction with life.

I'll miss words, and more important, I'll miss the feelings they trigger and the nuances of life they describe. I'm definitely passing out more words in the immediate future.

---

"Go away. I'm all right." The last six words of H.G. Wells. He was an English writer and social theorist. One of his time's most influential writers, he, along with Jules Verne, is credited with inventing the genre of science fiction. His best known novels, *The Invisible Man, The Time Machine,* and *War of the Worlds* are still read frequently today, and his one-volume history of the world is recognized as the best ever compiled by a single author.

*http://www.geocities.com/Athens/Acropolis/6537/real-w.htm*

# Back to the Future

Yesterday, a physician friend of mine asked me if I would join him in speaking to the American College of Physicians. Of course, I jumped at the opportunity. It is a personal goal of mine to show them one of the newly discovered faces of Alzheimer's disease—early-onset, early stage—to as many physicians as I can before I lose the ability to communicate effectively with them. Later in the day, he sent me an e-mail confirming my acceptance and noted the place, date, and time of the presentation. The date of the presentation was eight months after his request that I join him.

He thanked me for my interest and then cautioned, "I want you to be on the program. Perhaps we should wait until closer to the date to officially accept."

And there was Dr. Alzheimer, throwing *another* glass of cold water in my face! I always know I have Alzheimer's disease. I never questioned the diagnosis—well, maybe not *never,* but I now accept it as much as I believe I can or will. But the words, "perhaps we should wait until closer to the date" again reminded me. Perhaps how I feel and am today will not be how I feel and am eight months from today. Wow! Even with my retrieval problems, my inability to recall recent events, and all the other nicks and slices in my brain, I have not learned to adjust. Given the sinking feeling in my stomach, the knot in my throat, and the general malaise I quickly slipped into, it is apparent I have yet to learn to fully accept the immutable fact: *I have Alzheimer's disease.*

It is apparent that somewhere inside, I am wishing that this disease would suddenly stop advancing on my brain. I would like a "stand in place"—a freeze of my symptoms. I know there is no cure, but could there at least be a pause? Will I ever fully accept the truth?

# FAQs and FGAs

Enter *FAQ* into the Internet search engine Google and you will get more than one trillion, one-hundred and fifty million (1,150,000,000) responses. Who invented the term *FAQ?* What are *Frequently Asked Questions?* Who asks them? How frequently must they be asked to be considered FAQs, and who must ask them and who counts them? And what about answers? I have never seen FGAs (Frequently Given Answers to the FAQs) for those of us living with and in Alzheimer's disease!

From the mind and the heart of someone who has Alzheimer's disease, there are lots of questions and very few answers. Many of my questions must rise to the level of FAQs, at least among those in the population who share my diagnosis. Few come with FGAs.

"Why do you ask so many questions in your writings, and answer so few?" readers have asked.

One reason I don't offer answers is because I have lost much of my old self-confidence to solve my own problems. I don't have the problem-solving tools I once possessed: recall, language facilitation, a curiosity about most everything, an interest in learning as much as possible.

People around me have learned from their own personal experiences with me that I can't be trusted in the same ways they trusted me in the past. I misunderstand. I forget. Sometimes it goes beyond forgetting and misunderstanding: I'm bewildered about a world I once understood in the same way that others understood it. Why on earth would I look to myself—why on earth would others look to me—for answers?

I have more questions than usual because for me, each day, each week, each month is perceivably, and according to those around me impercep-tibly, different. Answers to the questions that make it easier for people to love each other don't seem to be working. How do we trust each other? What do we do when one of us seems "mad"? What are

> *I don't have the problem-solving tools I once possessed: re-call, language facili-tation, a curiosity about most everything, an interest in learning as much as possible.*

29

our faults? Our strengths? What do we talk about? What don't we talk about? Who handles what problems? How do they do it?

My family spent years stumbling across touchy questions and developing agreed-upon answers. What do we say when someone is putting on weight? What about when someone makes a mistake? Gets mad at someone? Feels in the mood (or not) for sex? Gets low marks on a report card? Feels lonely? What do we do or say to answer the unstated questions families ask each other every day? For some reason(s), the answers don't seem to be working as well as they did in the past. A whole new set of questions has changed the priorities of our FAQs and FGAs. Now, we don't focus as much on others as on ourselves. When will I find the time? How can I do this when I never did it before? Who will take care of me? How will I pay the bills? Questions and answers about showing commitment, love, and support for each other have been replaced by *lower-order needs* (as Abraham Maslow would observe).

The more I look inward, the more questions I have, and the fewer answers I seem able to produce. The more I lose my independence and consequently the more dependent I grow on others, the more questions and fewer answers I have. Because of the nature of the disease, I am now limited in what I learn from firsthand experience. There is little time for trial and error and trying again. Another question and problem has presented itself.

Who determines and defines the FAQs of Alzheimer's? Who has the true FGAs? No one has ever recovered from the disease and written a book or appeared on Oprah with answers based on personal experience. Some caregivers have written very personal diaries. Most of these diaries conclude with the realization that what worked for them would not necessarily work for others.

For most caregivers and individuals diagnosed with Alzheimer's disease, answers are proclaimed by health care professionals, some of whom have treated dozens and sometimes hundreds of individuals whose lives, relationships, finances, and futures have been redefined by the presence of Alzheimer's disease.

There are checklists, books, tapes, seminars, study groups, web sites, and on and on and on. Each and all of these offer answers. Most of these answers are directed to the questions of caregivers. Very few of the answers claim to answer the questions of individuals living with the diagnosis. *The fact is, most experts spend more time talking to and listening to caregivers than they do talking to and listening to those of us with dementia.* Some days, I'm not easy to talk to. Most days, I'm not easy to listen to. I have an ability to say in a thousand words what many other people could say in 10 words. That isn't to say I'm not funny, clever, interesting, and worth listening to. It's just a fact that, even on good days, I talk too much.

Answers to my questions which are provided by others sound and feel to me like the answerer didn't understand my question. Most people offer answers to their own questions, not mine. My questions, when answered by others, sound and feel to me as if people are avoiding my concerns and concentrating on their own "issues."

Perhaps too much time is spent trying to answer and question each other, when what I really need is to feel like I am being heard. I know you don't have all the answers. You also don't have all the questions! Neither do I! And the unanswered and sometimes unanswerable questions keep coming and coming with each new symptom of the disease.

I realize I sometimes do not make sense when I open my mouth and out comes a string of words, each of which is understandable, but when placed next to each other it is hard to figure out what the hell I'm talking about. My mind wanders, a lot. More and more I start talking about things I was thinking about, but we weren't necessarily talking about them at the time. I don't appreciate context as I did in the past. I blurt things out that are true, but everyone sees them as a "blurt" because I say them in the wrong context, or I say them at the wrong time or the wrong place or in the wrong way! I talk about topics of conversation we had hours or days or weeks

> *I know you don't have all the answers. You also don't have all the questions! Neither do I!*

ago as if we were in the midst of that conversation right now. If you think it's confusing to you when I speak this way, consider how confusing it is to me when you don't seem to understand what I am saying or appreciate the context in which it was said—at least the context between my ears.

I am increasingly sensitive about myself. If people dare ask me a question, or appear not to understand me, I become defensive: "What do you mean you don't know what I mean? How many times do I have to tell you?" I wince when others say these things to me, but I don't give them the same permission. In the old days, I said what I meant (and thought) and most times I meant what I said. If people didn't understand me, I said it again. If they still didn't understand me I made up an analogy and repeated it in different words an additional time. Now, if they don't seem to get it, I become frustrated. I'm not sure if I'm frustrated with having the disease, with the consequences of the disease, or with my apparent lack of perfection as a communicator!

What I currently seem best at and have the most need to do is to ask questions of myself, my caregivers, my physicians, my disease, and the U.S. Government. I guess when you're feeling scared and out of control, you have a lot of questions and very few answers. When the answers I receive come from individuals who are neither scared nor out of control in the way(s) I am, it is understandable why I feel a disconnect.

People sincerely tell me what's best for me. I know I don't always know what is best for me. Knowing that I am fallible does not in my mind automatically make the answerers infallible. Someone needs to sit down and straighten out the FAQs and FGAs for this disease, especially for those of us who have it.

I know I haven't been very successful thus far!

---

I once heard a physician say that 95% of success in a medical diagnosis comes from getting accurate information during the medical interview. Information comes from seeing, of course, but also from hearing what the other person has to say. And hearing is related to talking—asking the right questions based on what is heard.

*http://itre.cis.upenn.edu/~myl/languagelog/archives/003034.html*

# Alzheimer's Disease, Suicide, and Death

*The death of what's dead is the birth of what's living.*
—Arlo Guthrie

It would be intellectually dishonest to proclaim that I have never thought about suicide since being diagnosed with Alzheimer's disease. I have not pondered my own actual suicide, but I have considered pondering my own suicide. Is thinking about thinking about suicide the same as thinking about suicide? There is a very practical explanation as to why individuals with end-stage Alzheimer's do not take their own lives, nor do they ponder or plan the act. They simply lack the intellectual capacity, and the physical ability, to end their lives. However, what are individuals diagnosed with the disease to think when they are staring at a video of an individual in the end stage of Alzheimer's? What are we to think as we stare down the gun barrel of death, but have yet to crawl into it?

When first confronted with the reality of my Alzheimer's diagnosis, my mind jumped to the inevitable outcome of Alzheimer's disease: death. Death does not result from the disease itself but from one of the consequences of the disease. Respiratory failure can occur when a diseased mind forgets how to breathe. Organs forget what to do, how to cooperate, and how to clean themselves.

Life, death, living wills, powers of attorney—these all suddenly became very, very important to me. Especially my death! For a brief period of time, I was listening for just the right songs to play at my own memorial service. My first living will was more like a death will. It contained pages of instructions and suggestions to my caregivers on how best to care for me after I had passed on, or passed over, or passed out. I knew I was probably going to die with a whimper, but I wanted to go out with a bang!

It's amazing to me that when I discovered I had less control over my life than I had previously assumed, I promptly switched the focus of my energies to controlling the end of my life and circumstances

*For a brief period of time, I was listening for just the right songs to play at my own memorial service.*

after I was dead—a situation about which I could clearly exercise zero control.

Thus far, I feel I have lived a reasonably full and productive life. I have had my unproductive moments, days, months, and, at least once, years, but overall, I have done a pretty good job of living. From time to time, I realize that I have not fully let go of the folly of youth, thinking that I would live forever. Sometimes, especially when I make a commitment to somebody for some future activity, I pause and wonder if I will be able to honor this commitment. I think of friends I know and have known who wrestle with Alzheimer's, and I can measure their decline in days, weeks, and months better than I can measure my own decline. If this or that happened to them over the course of six months, will it happen to me? And when will those six months begin?

My current concerns about Alzheimer's and death focus not on the moment when my brain waves go flat, my heart ceases to beat, and I draw no more air into my lungs. The death I currently ponder does not have an on/off switch. It occurs in the months and perhaps years when I drift between consciousness of my current self and a consciousness of . . . I know not what. For me, this is the real death of Alzheimer's disease. Like a patient who lapses in and out of a coma, death comes and goes many times. What is it like to live, or die, like that? Lots of people know, but they cannot tell me.

There is a site on the Web I discovered that claims to be able to predict the exact day on which you will die. The Death Clock (www.deathclock.com): According to the formula on this Web site, I will die on November 16, 2016. If Alzheimer's (on average) reduces the average life span by 10 years, I should have died on November 16, 2006! Thank heaven there is no such person as Mr. Average.

# What Is It Like to Have Alzheimer's Disease—Three Years Later

It is now about three years since my daughter observed that "something is wrong with Dad." I have now lived with the diagnosis of Alzheimer's disease for about two years. Last year, about this time, I wrote "What Is It Like to Have Alzheimer's?" This is the second installment of that chapter.

Sometimes, when I am alone with my thoughts, I wander aimlessly around the corridors of my mind. I open various doors to see if they are still full of the memories I stored there long ago. To my pleasant surprise, most of them seem to contain all that I remember putting in the room. However, as I move from the past toward the present, I find more and more empty rooms. Not only are they empty, they are dark. They offer no clue, other than the label on the door, as to what they once contained.

And so in conversations, and private moments of thought, and sometimes just trying to get through the day, I open a door and it is dark. I have no clue what I stored in there. On some doors the lettering is faint, and on other doors the lettering has fallen off. The rooms are there but the contents are jumbled up, incomplete, difficult to make out, or sometimes just plain missing. It is very unnerving to be in the midst of a conversation and all of a sudden need to open the door to a room to access its contents and—the room is dark. I don't have a clue. – *My youngest granddaughter's name – Where I parked the car – If I parked the car – What I was talking about – What you were talking about – Where I was going – What I was doing –* What I am doing and what I have done!

I pause in my conversation and search for clues and connections. I race up and down the corridors of my mind, frantically seeking to make sense of what's going on around me. Sometimes this process makes

> *I race up and down the corridors of my mind, frantically seeking to make sense of what's going on around me. Sometimes this process makes me even more lost, and I become lost about why I am lost!*

me even more lost, and I become lost about why I am lost! I don't know what's going on because I come to an empty room, the dead end of a corridor, or I am on an unfamiliar floor of my mind. I am forced to pause and try to recall why I am here, but the blank doors around me give me no clues. My face takes on a quizzical look and sometimes I act embarrassed because I am lost.

I am no longer an observer of Alzheimer's disease. I am an unwilling participant in its process.

Yesterday, someone pointed out to me an incident of my confusion they witnessed, and I had no recollection of it. I think that was a preview of my next years of having Alzheimer's disease.

## TIPS FOR COMMUNICATING WITH A
## PERSON WHO HAS ALZHEIMER'S DISEASE

What can you do to help?

**Make allowances.** Try to remember that your loved one is not acting this way on purpose. Try not to take it personally. It's the disease talking, not your loved one.

**Show interest.** Maintain eye contact and stay near your loved one, so he or she will know you're listening and trying to understand.

**Avoid distractions and noise.** Communication is difficult, if not impossible, against a background of competing sights and sounds.

**Keep things simple.** Use short sentences and plain words. Avoid complicated questions or directions.

**Don't interrupt.** It may take several minutes for your loved one to respond. Avoid criticizing, hurrying, correcting and arguing.

**Don't raise your voice.** The disease affects the ability to concentrate, not to hear.

*http://www.mayoclinic.com/health/alzheimers/AZ00004*

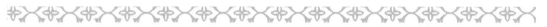

# Four No Trump

I am always looking for exercises to keep sharp or to sharpen whatever is left of my memory and executive function. I play an electronic game called Simon several times a day. I spend at least an hour a day at several sites on the Internet playing word and memory games. Some people work crossword puzzles and others read the paper. Over the past two years, I could have charted the uneven and inexorable deterioration of my cognitive abilities by how well I succeeded at these various games.

I am part of a study at a large medical school that provides a quarterly neuropsychological battery of tests. I spend about eight hours over two days tapping my fingers, remembering and repeating lists of words, telling the examiner who is the President of the United States, and answering other questions that seem important to him. I sometimes have trouble focusing my concentration or finding all the *w*s and *9*s in rows of letters and numbers, or pressing the space bar when I see an *X* preceded by an *A*. Every six months they show me five color charts and graphs comparing my scores across time.

I was told I should expect to fail parts of these tests. I should expect not to complete most of them. That is the way they are designed. Imagine someone who is unsure of his mental capacity prior to testing being told to relax because failure of these tests was no indication of mental capacity.

> "Hurry up," says the examiner, "but don't expect to finish."
> "Why hurry in the first place?" ask I.
> "Don't worry if you don't know all the answers," says the examiner.
> "Which ones is it okay for me to not know?" ask I.

Understand, there are no accepted norms for people with Alzheimer's on these tests. There is no agreement on the exact number of stages of the disease. There is no agreement on how long each stage lasts. There is no agreement on how to measure within stages or between stages. There is no agreement as to when and how fast any one individual should lose his or her cognitive functions. We can't even agree on the claim that as we grow older, we forget! We may remember, but we just can't recall it! But I do understand we have to start somewhere.

*"Don't worry if you don't know all the answers," says the examiner.*

I propose that all adults 30 years or older visit a neurologist once every three years. At that visit, they should play four games of duplicate bridge with the neurologist, or perhaps a new health care technician I will call licensed *Bridgeologists* (who will be entitled to place the initials *B.O.* after their names). Tape the game, and three years later when you return, play the identical hand again and videotape it. Compare games and scores. Did you count the same number of points? Did you play the hand the same way? Did you complete a finesse? Did you correctly count cards? Did you make the same score?

When I was a smart-ass undergraduate college debater, I started to play bridge. Of course, like most self-improvement efforts of male college-age youth, I did it to spend more time with a young lady whose attention I coveted. She was always a better bridge player than I, but I did win her heart—at least for a couple of years. Bridge teaches you to count the number of cards played in each suit. It teaches you to analyze the bidding of each of the other players and make assumptions about what is in their

*"Which ones is it okay for me to not know?" ask I.*

hands based on their bidding. Your executive function in your hippocampus is very, very busy during a bridge game. Your Golden Retrievers are running all over your brain fetching information.

Several years ago, I returned to bridge, playing with my computer. Now my opponents and partner are not psycho/social/sexual distractions or motivators, because only God and the other player know for sure the real age, sex, disposition, and sexual orientation of my partner and opponents.

At first I felt as if I was my old self, "The Iron Duke." Soon I saw that the Duke was more than just rusty. I started to play what I termed *assisted bridge*. I cheated, and next to me I kept the count of the cards, the suits, and the bidding on a 3×5 note card.

Now as I bid and play the hands, I can actually see evidence of the failure of my executive function to organize and understand information. I play some tricks which I know I should have won, and I haven't a clue as to why I failed to win the trick; I only know that I screwed up, but I can't understand why or how. I go back and replay

> *Perhaps playing bridge is easier, more cost-effective, accurate, and quicker than eight hours of neuro-psychological testing to measure the progress of the disease.*

the hand, and parts of it are still a mystery to me. Sometimes I don't follow suit. When the computer corrects me, I still don't follow suit. I'm looking at the hand and I electronically throw out the wrong suit, not once—sometimes twice!

I still know how to play bridge! I know the rules. I know the "tricks" of the game. I only have to count up to 13 cards in each of four suits and the games take no more than 5 or 10 minutes to play.

Perhaps playing bridge is easier, more cost-effective, accurate, and quicker than eight hours of neuropsychological testing to measure the progress of the disease. Perhaps, rather than ruling out every other disease known to medical students in order to get to an Alzheimer's diagnosis, half an hour of bridge every three years could be as accurate in diagnosing early-stage Alzheimer's.

It is an idea worthy of a double-blind, placebo-controlled, long-term, cross-cultural, cross-generational, longitudinal study. Don't you think? Just like they do with the pills and with me!!

There are several free and some subscription-based sites available for playing bridge on the Internet. OKBridge (www.okbridge.com) is the oldest of the still-running Internet bridge services; players of all standards, from beginners to world champions, may be found playing there. SWAN Games (http://www.swangames.com/main/index.html) is a more recent competitor. Bridge Base Online (http://www.bridgebaseonline.com/) is free, although options to earn masterpoints and play for money require prepayment. MSN and Yahoo!Games have several online Rubber Bridge rooms.

# "We Have a Pill.
# Alzheimer's Can Be Treated!"

*At this time, there is no medical treatment to cure or stop
the progression of Alzheimer's disease. FDA-approved
drugs may temporarily improve or stabilize memory
and thinking skills in some individuals.*
—http://www.alz.org/AboutAD/Myths.asp

On four different occasions, four different doctors (Yes, I know, I've seen a lot of doctors. Yes, I know, I frequently change doctors. Yes, I know, I frequently change insurance carriers. I make these changes as many times as my primary caregiver's employer changes insurance providers) have told me: "I have good news for you. At long last, we can treat Alzheimer's disease: We have a pill. We have something that can help you." And then in a slightly softer and less upbeat voice, one of them said: "Of course, it doesn't help everyone, and I make no guarantees, but for many of my patients this new family of drugs temporarily slows down the impact of the disease on your daily living." And then in even more hushed tones: "It does not stop or even slow down the disease; it appears to only delay the onset of some of the effects of the disease. Once it has lost its effectiveness, you will end up in the same place as those who have not taken the pill." Various studies of these drugs report that they have "helped" people for periods of time ranging from six months to two or perhaps three years to improve their "quality of life," their "daily living," their scores on this or that test, the perception of their caregivers' perception of them.

Recently, physicians have concluded that the drug may still be "helping" individuals in the second and third stages of Alzheimer's. They point to the fact that when some individuals abruptly stop using one of these drugs when they are in Stage 2 or 3, they exhibit a marked deterioration in their condition. It may be that the drugs have a noticeable impact on the disease for a brief period and imperceptibly slow down its progress for the rest of the person's life.

Having addressed some or all of these issues, each of the physicians smiled at me, wrote me a prescription for one of the drugs, and left the room.

One doctor paused at the door and turned to my wife and said: "You need not come back to see me until he pulls down his pants and pisses in the middle of the living room." The other three seemed quite content that they had done something for me, and other than offering to treat the inevitable depression and anxiety which seems to have bonded with this disease, this pill was their best shot.

Taking the long view of the history and treatment of Alzheimer's, I am sure it is reassuring to physicians, who in the past had to tell patients there was nothing they could do, to feel the sense of genuine pride and satisfaction that they now have a pill to offer us.

Assume I was in a serious automobile accident, and I awoke to hear my doctor saying to me:

> I have good news for you. The gear shift lever sticking out of your head will not be the cause of your death. Unfortunately, you will eventually bleed to death, and that process takes on average 10 years. The last two or three years of your life will be very difficult on you and your loved ones.
>
> The good news is I have a pill that for some people for some time, ranging from six months to two or three years, clots some of your blood and slows down the process. Unfortunately, the blood will simply build up behind the clot, and once the clot dissolves, you will lose the same amount of blood you would have lost up to that point had you not taken the clotting pill. As your physician, I am happy for you that I can offer this medication.

What should be an appropriate response from yours truly?

These pills seem to be seen from three different views: the physician, the caregiver, and the patient.

For physicians, once the diagnosis of Alzheimer's disease is made, confirmed, and announced, there is little or nothing more they can do to treat the patient. They wait for something to happen as a result of the disease—depression, anxiety, inappropriate behavior, problems with breathing and swallowing—and then treat the consequences of the disease with more pills. From their perspective, I am sure this pill feels better to them than saying, "I can't offer you an explanation of the disease, or a confident prediction of how and how much longer the patient will live. All I can say is 'I will do no harm myself to the patient.'"

And, in fact, one physician with whom I spoke was taken aback that I did not receive his news of the existence of this pill with a smile in my heart and a hardy handshake for him and the drug companies.

For caregivers, the pill is a godsend, sort of. It offers immediate relief, or at least the possibility of temporary relief, from living a life that they fear more than the disease itself. A recent survey revealed that the public at large and caregivers for individuals diagnosed with Alzheimer's fear being responsible for someone with the disease more than they fear actually having the disease themselves. For caregivers, the pill provides some factual basis to their hope that a cure will be found in time to help their loved one. After all, you don't go to the doctor for advice, you go to the doctor for a pill. Roots, fruits, and exercise don't cure diseases— pills do. If you are sad and don't want to be, take a pill. If you want to be happier, take a pill, or quicker yet, snort one, or the quick-est of all is to inject it right into a vein. Pills, pills, pills . . . are we not currently paying much, much more for them than they cost to make so that the struggling drug companies will have a few bucks left over to invent more pills?

> *One physician with whom I spoke was taken aback that I did not receive his news of the existence of this pill with a smile in my heart and a hardy hand-shake for him and the drug companies.*

It is not that I don't have questions about pills: Have you got it in a time-release form so I don't have to take a pill every three or four hours? Is it covered by my insurance? Can you treat the side effects with another pill? Is it habit-forming? Is there a generic for it? Can I buy it cheaper in Mexico or Canada? And my own personal favorite: Will it constipate me?

Pills provide new flimsy hooks that caregivers can hang on to when they feel the need to support their diminishing hope that a cure will be found. If only everyone can hang on to something long enough until the magic bullet is discovered!

For me, the pill sounded like good news, sort of. I read the stud-ies on which the claims and carefully worded advertisements were based. As new studies came out, studies not conducted by the owners of the pills or their well-financed panels, some of the colors of some of the pills started to fade. As I looked at the standards used to measure the effectiveness of the pills, some of them started to crack. As I tried to look at my own behavior, and listened to some of the exaggerated claims for the pills from others taking them, I questioned myself as to why I was taking them. Now I am in a quandary. I know I have passed the point where the pills could do/should do/did do me some good. I know the disease has and is progressing. I have scared myself into continuing to take the pills until the day before my death for fear that they are holding back some rush of ill-defined negative consequences to my mind. I have heard the stories of individuals stopping the pills for whatever reasons, quickly deteriorating, restarting the pills, and never recovering to where they were when they stopped.

For folks with serious depression, many of them go through a stage where they really, really appreciate pills that mess with the chemistry of their brains. Although no one can tell them exactly what is going on and why it is having the effect it has on their thinking, it beats what they had to deal with. Eventually they are forced to deal with the side effects of the chemistry experiments taking place in their minds. It turns out that, like in life, so too in brain chemistry experiments. There are trade-offs for everything. There are unintended consequences. Smart people, well-educated, well-intended, and on whose opinions we are encouraged to rely, make mistakes—mistakes that are only apparent with the benefit of hindsight.

Right now, I'm not sure if pills are good or bad news for me. However, they seem to make everyone else around me feel good. "May I please have a glass of water and another handful of pills?"

Popular literature in the late 1970s asserted that Americans were "overmedicated." Writers emphasized the drugs' addictive potential, aggressive promotion by drug manufacturers, and irresponsible prescribing by physicians, concluding that millions of people were—or were likely to become—addicted. Although many drug use and prescription studies, and much clinical experience, failed to support the idea of an overmedication threat, this information was largely ignored. The overmedication construct persisted because it helped Americans express disillusionment with medical care and fears about a complex and changing world. It simplified reality and created villains and victims, helping to shape an agenda for reform. . . . This historical study demonstrates that risk perception is guided as much by cultural beliefs and values as by information, and implies that, regardless of available scientific knowledge, enduring drug myths have helped determine American drug policy since 1900.

*http://repository.upenn.edu/dissertations/AAI9308663/*

# Dreams, Drugs, Alzheimer's, and Me

*. . . side effects can include leg cramps, nausea, vomiting, constipation or diarrhea; problems falling asleep or waking up; patients will have more vivid dreams; they may have nightmares . . .*

—Paraphrasing almost every drug pamphlet in existence

When you dream, and by the way we all do dream, the front part of your brain attempts to disconnect itself from the core of your brain. The core experiences a thunderstorm of electrical activity during specific times in the sleep cycle. Occasionally, some of this electrical activity leaks into the front of the resting part of your brain.

> "What does this mean? This stimulation must mean something. Can't see, can't hear, can't feel. I've got to figure this out," says your frontal lobe to itself. Let the dreams begin! "Ooops, what are these chemicals doing to my natural dream process? I would think that after 61 years of trying to figure out and get control of his dreams, he would leave well enough alone and just let me figure this out," says the frontal lobe to the hippocampus. "But no, just because he was feeling a little down, he starts swallowing pills that stimulate me in ways I have no control over. I don't like what's going on," complains the frontal lobe. "I'll show him what happens when he changes pills . . . "

Last night I was in Bosnia, riding through war-torn villages on top of a tank! The night before last, I was in Botswana, riding along in a Jeep through open countryside! Who knows where I will be tonight? I have started to recall my dreams. I have started to have "lucid" dreams: I am aware I am dreaming, but it feels like I am a part of the dream.

I have changed my medications!

Messing around with drugs that mess around with dopamine, and the various receptors between my ears that drink the stuff, almost always causes me problems with my dreams. We all dream. We all do not recall all our dreams. Some nights, we recall more dreams than other nights.

I do not like to dream (that is to say, I do not like to recall my dreams). I would rather close my eyes at midnight and open them at 8:00 A.M., remembering nothing of what happened inside or outside my head during the night. Pre-Alzheimer's, I was blessed with a brain chemistry that didn't quite put my frontal lobe to sleep in REM (the rapid eye movement state of sleep), so while I was dreaming I was aware enough that I realized I was dreaming while I was dreaming. These are lucid dreams.

It has been six months since last I looked at the contents of my morning and nightly drug cocktail. I believe it should be looked at every six months through my eyes, the eyes of my caregivers, the eyes of a neurologist, gerontologist, family care physician, psychologist, psychiatrist, and any others looking into my health at the moment, who I believe might see something I can't.

We do not have a time line for the progression of Alzheimer's disease. For me it seems to advance in spurts, with unequal periods of time in between the spikes of activity. I try to look at myself from the inside out, while the professionals look at me from the outside in. Sometimes these different perspectives result in different conclusions concerning what to change and what not to change in my daily handful of pills. If most of the committee agrees that nothing much seems to have changed, I move that we continue my current drug protocols (code of conduct), my spouse seconds it, I call for the vote, it is usually unanimous, we make a new appointment in six months, we pay everyone at the table a co-pay, and we leave.

If something seems to have changed, we discuss it, look for ways address the change, and change what we believe needs to be changed. Most times, these changes concern the drugs I consume with breakfast and dinner. "Take more, take less, take this, take that, and don't forget you should never drink grapefruit juice," say the seers seated around the conference table. I go home and throw

> *If most of the committee agree that nothing much seems to have changed, I move that we continue my current drug protocols, my spouse seconds it, I call for the vote, it is usually unanimous, we make a new appointment in six months, we pay everyone at the table a co-pay, and we leave.*

out perfectly good (and expensive) drugs, and I fill more and different prescriptions.

That very night, I start to become a participant in my dreams. They seem like real experiences because I can feel them. They are dreams because I can think about myself while I am feeling the dream. I wake up still feeling them. I wake up wondering how I can be so worked up over a dream. I wake up wishing I didn't remember my dreams. I wake up and it is one day closer to reexamining my drug protocols.

It is bad enough having to live with forgetting. It is even worse when what you can remember causes additional distress!

Everyone seems to agree there is nothing that can be done to halt Alzheimer's disease because no one knows the cause. Why is it that everyone, primarily psychiatrists and neurologists (you *know* they are attached at the brain during medical school and are only surgically detached when they go into their residencies), prescribes pills to deal with the side effects of other pills which deal with the side effects of the disease? My brain is already in open rebellion to the "normal" ways of processing and storing information.

Perhaps I need to hold fewer pill conferences and more "me" conferences. I need to pay better attention to me and trust my brain to take care of the rest.

# I Wish I Were a Nude Mouse

Almost daily, I read of some group of nude mice being cured of some horrible disease. Recently, I have seen articles about nude mice with variations of Alzheimer's disease. When these mice were given this or that chemical, they were cured of the element of Alzheimer's disease with which they were afflicted.

If we can do it for mice, surely we can do it for humans. Miroslav Holub, a Czech immunologist, and a very famous poet in his time, was the first person to discover and identify a nude mouse. How it happened—the nude mouse, that is—has not to my knowledge been documented. I do know he began to breed them and was soon able to pursue poetry full time because he made so much money from the sale of nude mice.

The reality is that a nude mouse is a mutant mouse (http://www.medterms.com/script/main/art.asp?articlekey=33771). It is called a *nude* mouse, first, because it is hairless, and second, because it has two copies of the gene called *nu*. It is homozygous for the recessive mutant *nu* gene. (I will bet you could not learn this watching *American Idol*.)

In addition to qualifying for the tax exemptions and other special benefits given to nude mice (tax credits and depreciation for certain modifications they had to make to their cages to assist themselves to safely take a bath, use the restroom, and get in and out of bed), you must have been born without a thymus gland. If you are any form of animal and don't have a thymus at birth, unfortunately you have no capacity to make T-cells, a class of lymphocytes which swim around in our blood and seek out and destroy foreign invaders. Without T-cells, you cannot reject tumors or tissues from other animals, and your immune system is not worth two cents.

Perhaps being a nude mouse isn't all that it seems to be at first sniff. The jump in science from a two-ounce nude mouse to 220-pound yours truly is truly a quantum leap. A "cure," for me, is to continue to collect the bits and pieces we are learning about the disease and see if they will "fit" into my life. Personally, I believe it will be a long, long time before we understand the disease process and all its causes. As with AIDS treatments, I think the next breakthrough in treating my disease will be the development of pharmacological cocktails flavored to meet the tastes of individual drinkers. We need to get over the "take this pill and come back when I can treat some of the side effects of the disease" mentality prevalent in some physicians today.

I have stopped reading about the "breakthroughs" in research on Alzheimer's disease that appear so frequently in the popular press. If they find what causes it, how to stop it, how to reverse the damage it causes to healthy brains, then I'll buy the special issue of *Time* magazine and read it. Until then, I read the medical journals for Alzheimer's disease studies that produce statistically significant results as measured by some set of questions, or some pre- and postobservations by a caregiver. Should I take more or less of vitamins E, B, and C and folic acid? Should I beg for immunotherapy, ignoring the risks and concentrating on the five people who did so well when they underwent it? What about lowering my cholesterol and my blood pressure? I already eat lots of broccoli.

> *I have stopped reading about the "breakthroughs" in research on Alzheimer's disease that appear so frequently in the popular press.*

Unfortunately, I am not, never was, and never will be a nude mouse. On balance, I'm still glad to be who I was, who I am, and who I will be.

There are 398,000,000 Web listings for the word *mouse* in Google.

# "I Have Been Diagnosed with Alzheimer's Disease"

Whenever you have first-hand experience with something, you are sensitized to it in your surroundings. Break your arm and you will be amazed at how many people you know who have broken their arms. Buy a new home and lots and lots of people will tell you their home-buyers' stories. Discover you have cancer and almost everyone you know will know someone who had or has cancer and has a story to tell.

What happens when you tell people you have Alzheimer's disease? My experience has been that the announcement is initially met with silence. People then express their sorrow, mention something about an article they read about new advances in the fight against the disease, and then change the subject. The next time we meet, they apologize for not "saying more," and then with watery eyes they tell me their experience with the disease in a relative, friend, or neighbor.

I believe Alzheimer's has replaced cancer as the most feared disease people can imagine. Like cancer, there is really little we can do to avoid it. (Come on now, please, let's get real: "Eat more broccoli"?). There is no cure for Alzheimer's, and it asserts total control of your mind and eventually your body. The disease does what it wants with us and to us, and we are reduced to being observers of the demise of our own minds.

> *I believe Alzheimer's has replaced cancer as the most feared disease people can imagine.*

I admit, I don't have a more appropriate or supportive way of responding to the announcement of friends or family members who announce that they have been diagnosed with Alzheimer's disease. It was a shock to me when I first heard it, as it will be a shock to you when you hear it from someone else. We don't know much about it. Much of what we do "know" is not true or is only partly true. If we don't have it, we don't want to know much about it. We don't want to admit to ourselves that we need to know much about it. Out of sight, out of mind. It's the way I was living. It's the way I would still like to live.

# While Rome Burns . . . A Parable

Once upon a time, July 18, 64 A.D., to be exact, fire started to sweep through 10 of the 14 districts comprising the City of Rome. In these districts were the homes of mostly older Romans. Richard Tiberius Augustus Taylor was a 61-year-old psychology teacher who lived in one of those homes. When he heard that his home was threatened, he rushed to it. Running down the narrow, crooked streets of old Rome, he could feel the heat. Everyone seemed in a panic. Even the adult children of the residents didn't know what to do. The residents seemed bewildered and confused.

Upon arriving home, Richard and his neighbor, a neurophysiologist, surveyed the damage and found it to be minimal thus far. But Richard could still feel the heat. It was as if the fire was smoldering within him. He reached in his toga and pulled out his newly purchased cell phone. Dialing his local fire department, he knew they would be able to save him and his house. After redialing 10 times, someone finally answered.

"Sorry, Citizen Taylor, we are real busy here right now. A lot of people seem to be calling us about this fire," said the voice at the other end. "We don't know exactly what's going on, but as soon as we figure it out, you can bet, depending on the amount of fire coverage you purchased, we will be there to help you. Right now, we're suggesting all people threatened by the fire spread six months of retardant around the edge of their house. In many cases, this has been shown to slow the rate of the fire."

"My house is still going to burn down to the ground," Richard pleaded into the phone.

"We just don't know enough about this fire, or what kind of a fire it really is, to start throwing chemicals on it. We don't want to make it worse. You know our motto is 'Do no harm.' Right now, our hoses are tied."

"But my house is going to burn down!" an anxious and increasingly depressed Richard responded.

"I've heard there are some double-blind studies going on at the Firefighting Training Academy. You might call them and see if you can participate."

Richard called the Academy and spoke to the chief. "My house is burning down. How can you help me?"

The chief responded, "I'm glad you called. We have a number of ongoing studies, some as far as Phase 2 on fire prevention and fire retardants. I am very sorry, but that is the best the Academy can offer you right now. Unfortunately, we are not miracle workers."

"Don't you people understand?" said Richard. "The fire is already burning my house! I need someone to put it out, not prevent or retard a fire that's already consuming me. I am on fire! NOW!"

Over the course of the next six days, 60% of old Rome was reduced to ashes.

Tacitus, an aristocrat and historian, attempted to blame Emperor Nero for the fire. This parable is not about blame. It is not about who caused the fire. It is not about the fire department, who did not have access to the technology to fight the fire. It is about the citizens who perished in the fire, victims of being born in the wrong century.

> *Let's not fiddle around. Let's do what we can do today to support the victims, their caregivers, and the doctors.*

While Rome burns, let's not fiddle around. Let's do what we can do today to support the victims, their caregivers, and the doctors. Alzheimer's disease is burning up years and years of the productive, happy lives of millions of people.

"Help! I'm on fire!"

# Trying to Figure It Out

How does someone who has already exhibited the signs of plaque in his brain figure out what is going on between his ears? How do I understand understanding? How do I understand how I understand? How am I different from others? What difference does the difference make?

Trying to "figure out" Alzheimer's when you have Alzheimer's is like trying to figure out how to build the space shuttle from a set of plans written in 10 different languages which were dropped on the way over and just randomly reassembled. And oh, by the way, we were not sure if these are all the plans or the right plans because it would be unethical to test them using live human beings. Even on a good day, there is no one person on Earth who understands all it takes to build the space shuttle. It is so complicated that most of the problems that occur are compatibility issues (the right-hand engineer does not know or understand what the left-hand engineer is doing, so when the computer programs of each hand meet in the processor they produce error readings). Shuffle all the pages of their designs, and there is little if any use in reading beyond page one because the next page is not logically related to the previous page. In fact, logic and reason get in the way of understanding what is going on, because the pages are mixed up.

Some of my logic circuits are now misconnected. Some of them misfire in some circumstances and work in other circumstances. Some of them are just plain disconnected. Some of the information I fed into them was improperly entered. Some of the information was just made up. Some of the information is just plain missing. Yet I insist on trying to make sense of all this garbage in and garbage out. I try to understand what is going on with me. I try to predict what I will do, and when I will do it. I try to explain what I did and why I did it. I try to understand inconsistencies in my own behaviors, and explain why they were inconsistent with each other.

How can I do this "right" in the morning and "wrong" in the afternoon? Why do I recall details no one else remembers and forget major points everyone knows? There is a growing industry of professionals who are increasingly more accurate at explaining why people with Alzheimer's do what we do (maybe in a few small studies), but they have less success in predicting what we will do and under what circumstances we will do it. There are some behaviors they can predict, but those are usually from individuals in the later stages of the disease, when deteriorating physiology is more in control than psychology.

*How can I do this "right" in the morning and "wrong" in the afternoon? Why do I recall details no one else remembers and forget major points everyone knows?*

Caregivers, most of whom maintain the hope that we don't have Alzheimer's well past the point of reasonable doubt, point to inconsistencies in our behaviors—predictable versus unpredictable, normal versus abnormal, expected versus unexpected—and say, "See, I told you this isn't Alzheimer's. If you were really diseased, you would always act in a diseased way."

The truth is that we do not know near as much as we think we do about how and why the "normal" brain works. The fact that Freud was wrong in most of his conclusions (a conclusion drawn by yours truly and a few thousand others) does not cause us to pause and question the assumption that thinking about thinking can answer any questions we have about thinking. We are now guessing (albeit educated) at the relationship between brain activity and behavior. When we think about the color red, this part of the brain scan turns green. So?

We have some ideas. We have some tests. We have some medications that seem to change behavior by changing the chemistry in the brain. How or why they work is, again, a matter of speculation. We don't fully understand the chemistry in the first place. How can we figure out what is wrong when we can't explain what is right?

We know lots more about Alzheimer's than did Dr. Alzheimer, yet we still do not know what causes it. We still do not know why some people deteriorate rapidly and others take years. We do not know what we are doing relative to the agreed-upon big picture of how the brain works, because there is no big picture. We do know that we don't know enough yet to do anything about stopping it, reversing it, or keeping people from getting it in the first place. (This last claim remains unfortunately true even in the face of headlines reporting that researchers have discovered that doing this or that, or eating this or that, prevents Alzheimer's. *Nothing prevents Alzheimer's disease.*

What we don't know could fill more books than what we do know! So here I am, trying to figure it, and me, out. I do not have the benefit of studying more than one subject. I cannot stop the progress and concentrate on one stage. At best, I am looking through a cracked and smoked glass at myself. My caregivers are looking through "Coke bottle" glasses and a number of other filters. We ask each other "why this" and "what about that," and what we get in response from each other is, "Well, it's been my experience that. . . ." We ask doctors, and no two of them give us the same answer. Some give no answer, change the subject, and increase the dose of our medications.

What am I to do? I, who use information to calm my fears; I, who believe if only I could figure out what was happening and why, I would be less fearful; I, who want to know what is next for me.

I keep reading. I consult Mr./Ms. Google and two-hundred dozen of my favorite web sites. I talk with other passengers sailing with me on the *SS Alzheimer.* I watch them. I listen to them. I talk with them. Am I any closer to understanding what is going on inside of me? Maybe, sort of, sometimes: in reality, probably not! What's the use of going on like this? I do not know. It keeps my perpetually busy mind under control, sort of. It uses up time I could have spent enjoying the flowers or feeling sorry for myself.

Does it make sense? NO! But then, neither does Alzheimer's disease. I am Alzheimer's before Alzheimer's is fully me! Ironic, isn't it?

# Checking Back in During Intermission . . . What Is It Like to Have Alzheimer's?

This has to be one of the longest intermissions of my life! It started about a year ago, with the end of Act One of my Alzheimer's disease. I was afraid of Act Two because I heard I would be required to drift in and out, back and forth, from my old self to my new self. Playing two characters, both at the same time; I wasn't looking forward to being someone with two identities.

I admit that several times during this intermission, I have peeked through the mezzanine doors and have seen the actors, including my stand-in, rehearsing Act Two. It is an odd feeling to watch someone playing the part of you. You know they aren't you, but they are!

During this extended intermission, caregivers have pointed out to me a number of incidents during which I was unaware of what

> *I was afraid of Act Two because I heard I would be required to drift in and out, back and forth, from my old self to my new self.*

I was doing. Even more amazing to me, when told what I did, I didn't seem to care! And, as a matter of fact, I really don't feel like I should care right now. It doesn't make sense, but it is how I think and feel right now, nursing my Bloody Mary until Act Two begins. It is simply amazing to be aware of what you don't want to do, and when you do it, not to care one way or the other. . . . Am I turning into an android that really doesn't care where it is, what is happening around it, what is happening to it? I have wandered away and I didn't care, and I don't care, although it sure upset a lot of other people. I didn't get upset about it. I was not and still am not afraid. Others are upset and afraid for me.

As the intermission drags on and I continue to nurse my one watery Bloody Mary, I have noticed that I have developed the tendency to forget things that people tell me. I forget people's names. Twice, I have forgotten where the restroom is. I have lost track of the number of times I forgot to do something that I told somebody I would do. In the past, behavior like that would upset me. In the recent past, it would frustrate me. In the present, it just doesn't seem to bother me that much. Why are others around me so concerned? I forgot— so what?

And so, I wander about the lobby, waiting for the lights to flash to signal the start of Act Two. They have yet to flash, but they may be dimming. Maybe they don't flash to signal the start of Act Two; maybe they just slowly dim to the point where we cannot see each other in the lobby and everyone walks in and takes a seat, and Act Two begins without a musical prelude.

I don't know, and I don't much care one way or the other.

(I can't stand sipping watered-down tomato juice. I may have to order a tall gin and tonic, unless this show gets moving soon.)

# Volcanoes, Fears, and Alzheimer's Disease

T here are more than 1,500 active volcanoes in the world. A volcano is considered active if it has erupted at least once in the last 10,000 years!

There are more than 24 million individuals diagnosed with Alzheimer's in the world. Multiply that number by the average number of active caregivers for each diagnosed individual (2.7), and *64+ million* is the approximate number of individuals in this world who are living, breathing human volcanoes, fired not by the movement of their tectonic plates but by the fears fueled by the diagnosis of Alzheimer's disease.

The temperature of the magma within a volcano depends on the composition and age of the magma. It ranges from 700 °C to 1,100 °C. (For citizens of virtually the only developed country in the world that has not converted to the metric system, the temperature range is 1,292 °F to 2,012 °F.) The temperature of the magma is also influenced by how deep within Earth the liquid roots of the volcano reach and how close they are to the liquid core. The estimated temperature of Earth's core is 7,000 °C, or 12,632 °F.

> *64+ million is the approximate number of individuals in this world who are living, breathing human-volcanoes.*

Fear, the fears generated by Alzheimer's disease, behaves much like magma. It spends most of the time unseen, under the crust. Some fear runs deep into our inner being. When it bursts, it burns all in its path. It quickly hardens, with a crust that cannot be penetrated easily. When someone or something manages to break the crust, more fear rushes out to burn all in its path and then to crust over again.

Some individuals diagnosed with the disease, and some caregivers, are like volcanoes of fear. From a distance, they appear calm, holding it together, in control. The closer you get to them, the more you listen, the greater your powers of observation, the more you can sense the real situation.

There are intrusions and extrusions of magma. We never see the intrusions of magma, the fear-driven issues that shift around within the walls of the volcano and never erupt. The extrusions of fear rush through cracks in the walls of the volcano, flowing down its sides and threatening all in its path, especially those in close proximity.

Occasionally, observers climb to the top of active volcanoes to see what is going on inside. This is a very risky journey, and frequently when they reach the top, all they can see is crust, with an occasional vent hole erupting now and then.

I believe our fears, and specifically my fears—fear of losing control, fear of what will happen tomorrow, fear of who I will become, fear of the unknown, and the list goes on—are as much or more of a problem for me in my day-to-day living than is the disease itself.

I have volcanic moments, as do my caregivers. We are all in a field of volcanic activity which is maintained by the tectonic plates fired by Alzheimer's disease. We cannot move away from the field. We are like mountains stuck in the earth that surrounds us. We rumble at others, each other, and ourselves. When we erupt, we lose control of our ability to hold in all the heat-fear connected to the deep source of our fears at the center of our being. We do not have the time or the energy to deconstruct ourselves, pick up the pieces, and reconstruct ourselves in a healthier place; our lives and the earth are spinning too fast to move too far away from our centers.

> *We are like mountains stuck in the earth that surrounds us. We rumble at others, each other, and ourselves.*

I must do more than simply wear a T-shirt that says, "Beware of occasional eruptions of my fears of volcanic proportions." I am frustrated with people who continually tell me, "Well, that's the way I am. My mother was that way, her mom was that way, and I act that way." It's as if their historical account of how generations of family members have acted inappropriately was justification for them carrying on the family's traditions. If lots of people with Alzheimer's disease become defensive, does that make it okay for me? Does the explanation of inappropriate behavior serve as an excuse for it?

I think not. I am still just as responsible for myself whether my mom suffered from manic depression or lived a Mother Teresa life.

I submerge myself in the science of the disease in the hope it will insulate me from my own fears. It doesn't. I spend a lot of time trying to understand the disease process rather than trying to understand my own fear processes. I am, in fact, more fearful of my fears than I am of the disease! Understanding my fears, like understanding volcanoes, does nothing to get me out of harm's way during eruptions. I could spend 100 hours in therapy or 100 hours reading about volcanoes, and if I have Alzheimer's disease or live at the foot of a volcano I am still in just as much peril. I can't move the volcano, and I can't cure myself of Alzheimer's. Guess I better look inside myself and address my fears and why I insist on living at the foot of a volcano. The solutions are in me. The solutions are me.

# Hemingway, Alzheimer, and Taylor*

>XCXCXCXCX

*Every man's life ends the same way. It is only the details of how he lived and how he died that distinguish one man from another.*

—Ernest Hemingway

I am a lot like Ernest Hemingway. He had a gray beard and so do I. We both liked to fish. He enjoyed daiquiris; I enjoy daiquiris. (Late in life, Hemingway convinced himself he was a diabetic. He invented a daiquiri with no sugar but twice the rum! Google "mojito" to find his recipe.) We are also alike in other ways, except that I did not write about my lifelong search for the purpose of life.

We both began our lives as idealists searching for role models. With Hemingway, it was the writer Gertrude Stein. With me, it was my speech teacher, John Walsh, and the Chicago Seven (for details, Google "Chicago Seven").

Ernest wanted to grow to be like Gertrude; I wanted to grow to become like my heroes. As we both got to know our heroes, it turned out that they were not as perfect as we thought they were or as we wanted them to be. They didn't know it all. Their reason for being was not as pure or known to them as we wished. They didn't always practice in their own lives what they preached to others!

According to Hemingway and Taylor, many of their heroes lived for the wrong reasons! Disillusioned with their quest to find meaning in their own lives by copying others, they turned inward.

Hemingway wrote *The Old Man and the Sea,* and Taylor divorced his role model and became a high school teacher. (I will resist my urge to detail my interpretation of Santiago's [the old fisherman's] battle with the great fish, and how in the end the absence of his best and only friend Manolin reveals to the fisherman his need for approval and interaction with others.)

---

*Mostly for undergraduate and graduate English majors and my brother Robert Taylor, who himself was an English teacher for more than 20 years before he discovered that retirement was better than the administrivia, controls, and the culture of today's high schools.

Hemingway found fame and fortune, and a sense of living an unfulfilled life (when he was sober). Successful as a teacher and debate coach, Taylor found frustration and a deep existential loneliness. Although both were surrounded by relative success by others' standards, there was still an emptiness that embraced them at the deepest levels of their feelings.

If I could not find my purpose by copying others, and I could not find it in myself, where was it to be found? Relationships!

Hemingway wrote *Islands in the Stream,* a novel which closely parallels Hemingway's life and sort of hints at Taylor's. Taylor bounced around until moving to Houston, where he fell in love and married the love of his life, Linda. Blessed with two children, Taylor found these relationships invigorating and fulfilling. Both Taylor and Hemingway were confident they had at last found the key to self-actualization, a unique sense of self and purpose, and loving reciprocal relationships.

Taylor's children grew up. His son joined the Air Force and moved away. He married someone Taylor had not met prior to the wedding. His son had kids and lived 1,000 miles away, away from the influence and knowledge of Taylor. His family became their own selves—something he had encouraged and expected, but not always in the way it was happening.

I came across Dr. Alzheimer at a most inopportune time in my life. Still wrestling with my own *raison d'etre* ("reason for being," just in case you don't speak French), Alzheimer's started to scramble my brain, surely shortened my life, and presented the inevitability of a true nihilist life experience devoid of relationships and introspection. Personally, I don't believe there is a single, unique, one-size-fits-me purpose and meaning of my life. I believe life, the world, the universe just is. I make what I want and need of it. I am my own person. I am a piece of the meaningless universe. Therefore . . . You get it. I am the meaning of my life. My thinking creates me for me. While I am aware of others' perceptions of me, ultimately I either accept or reject those perceptions as being a part of who I am. For me, the meaning and purpose of my life is intertwined with relationships. It took me quite a while and quite a few relationships to fig-

> *Personally, I don't believe there is a single, unique, one-size-fits-me purpose and meaning of my life. I believe life, the world, the universe just is. I make what I want and need of it.*

ure that out. Currently, my present, my future, and my relationships are in turmoil, compliments of Alzheimer's disease. There are many, many external forces that overwhelm most human beings, which can't be resisted unless you are, or appear to be, a very special human being. Even Mother Teresa had her eccentricities which some would characterize as faults or sins. I know, I knew a long time ago, that I was not destined for sainthood. My task was to live a life that satisfied me. Satisfying me was, in part, a function of loving and satisfying others—a function of giving myself to others without expecting a return in kind. This is all easier said than done. The devil, of course, is in the details.

Nihilism, and the thought of dying, no longer frighten me. Most times in my life I've done my best—sometimes I have not. I have tried hard, most of the time, to live a purposeful life and include others in my purpose. I have lived, from my perspective, a full, active, and useful life. That is what I eventually ended up hoping for. Cognitive diseases complicate the end-of-life experience. No death bed conversions, no apparent bright lights, no goodbyes and sage advice to loved ones for me.

Most people seem happy with a lack of pain as the goal of dying with this disease. But the absence of pain is not a purpose. It is a desirable prerequisite to what? I wish I knew. I wish I could speculate on it. I cannot.

# *Waiting for. . .*

*Some have referred to* Waiting for Godot *as "the play where nothing happens." In reality, there is plenty to watch and enjoy. The lack of a conclusive plot or ending is only frustrating if we expect all lives to have definitive, preordained directions and conclusions. The truth is that we all drift through life looking for answers. We all wait and we all look to other forces to provide us with answers and direction. There is no mystical, subliminal message contained within* Waiting for Godot. *Beckett always said that ". . . it means what it says."*

—(http://72.14.207.104/search?q=cache:LIMeGEtilSkJ:www.rondotheatre.co.uk/production.php%3FID%3D52

+looking+for+godot&hl=en&gl=us&ct=clnk&cd=13)

When I first stumbled across Dr. Alzheimer in my brain, he was an occasional nuisance. He would empty a room full of memories here and there, and cause a couple of doors to stick, but I devised strategies to get around his tricks. Later, he became a frustrating pain in the ass. He would confuse my thought processes from time to time. I couldn't figure things out the way I had prior to meeting him. Now, he is a constant companion. Every day, every hour, every few minutes, I lose my train of thought. Not only do I lose it, I can't recall the name of the train, where I was going, or why I wanted to go there. Faces are merely familiar; the name is gone without leaving a trace. I am interrupted in my thought processes by improvised explosive devices left by Dr. Alzheimer. They explode between my ears but are not noticed by passers-by outside of my head. My life is an ongoing struggle to stay on track, to complete the thought, to find the right words, to hold myself together in the eyes of others when we are speaking. If a third person enters the conversation, I am simply lost. Now where was I? What were they saying? Conversations pass me by as I struggle to keep up, keep on track, and stay in the game.

> *I'm sure there is humor in my life, even now. I am sure there is unique meaning and purpose in my life, especially now.*

My fingers are losing contact with my brain, or vice versa. When I attempt to put pen to paper, or words to Word, there is a communication breakdown.

Like the tramps in *Waiting for Godot,* I stand around hoping something will happen, someone will come and straighten it all out. In the meantime, my life goes nowhere; there seems little purpose other than to simply wait and watch. I direct my struggles to hanging on to yesterday. I am missing today and don't even want to think about tomorrow.

I don't think Godot is ever going to show up. Where is the meaning, the purpose, the happiness in being me today? The longer I wait, the more limited my cognitive options seem to be. But who or what am I waiting for? Me? To get better? To stop getting worse?

I'm sure there is humor in my life, even now. I am sure there is unique meaning and purpose in my life, especially now. Maybe I shouldn't try so hard to find it; frustrate myself so much trying to understand it; disappoint myself so much trying to change it.

I'm going to try standing around for a while and see what it feels like, watch what happens. Maybe I should have done more of this in the past!

# Disabling Enablers

P ardon me if I whine a little. Aren't professionals supposed to help me? Aren't caregivers supposed to enable me to maintain a "normal" life as long as possible?

At best, the professionals who are on my team provide lists to my caregivers on how to keep me from hurting myself and others, when and how I should stop driving or handling money, and how to keep me from becoming lost in my own house or neighborhood. Professionals train caregivers how to cope with their own feelings and deal with me. Attention that is paid to people who have the disease frequently focuses on how to disable us so we won't harm ourselves and/or others.

At worst, the professionals who are on my team meet privately with my caregivers, who, in turn, air their complaints and frustrations about me and ask for suggestions on how they can improve their lives, mostly by improving my behaviors. The professionals become cheerleaders for caregivers, and sympathetic observers of me. The professionals are well-intentioned, but it is quicker and easier to "fix" caregivers than it is to listen to, understand, and even attempt to "fix" me. Caregivers' needs are clearer, more consistent, and easier to addresses than mine! My recollections of the past can't be trusted. What I want changes from day to day in ways others can't understand—and, for that matter, neither can I.

Where can I find the books on how I can live with my disease? How I can be enabled, not disabled, by my caregivers to truly be all that I can be at any given moment of my life, even with this disease? Clearly, the emphasis has been and is on the care and keeping of caregivers, and on discovering the causes of the disease (if it really is a single disease with one or more simple causes). I realize that if my caregivers are not around, or if they are depressed and anxious, then I receive less support and care. It is in my best interest to keep them in tip-top mental and physical shape. But, why not spend a bit more time and effort talking with people who have the disease? Studying our needs? Coming up with ideas to make our lives both safer and more fulfilling (and not necessarily in that order)? Why not spend less time with nude mice and more time with early-stage, early-onset folks?

Why not see us as a source of answers to our problems, rather than as a source of problems to which our caregivers need answers. We, too, want to be proactive when dealing with our symptoms, not just reactive to our problems!

Professionals, encourage caregivers to talk to us about their problems, and encourage them to listen to us about our problems. Cut down on the visits to you, and increase the time we spend around the kitchen table trying to solve our issues, not just theirs. Teach caregivers how to act as if our problems are real. You know, they are real to us! We try, in our own ways, to communicate. Honor us for trying. Don't tell us we are doing it the wrong way, or doing it in a manner you can't understand. Caregivers have far more flexibility in how they approach and solve problems than do we.

> *We try, in our own ways, to communicate. Honor us for trying.*

By their very nature (messing with our heads), the symptoms we label as *Alzheimer's disease* create as many or more psychological problems as they reflect physiological problems. At least for a while, there isn't much that can be done about what is happening with the chemistry between my ears, so why not spend more time working on what is happening to the chemistry between my spouse and me? Between mothers and daughters? Within families? Among friends?

For me, this is the neglected battle front of Alzheimer's disease. Just because we label it as a disease doesn't mean we can't react to it as if it were a cancer on marriage, a compound fracture between a father and his son. We don't have to wait for me to die to know for sure that fear of the future, fear of loss of self, fear of dying twice is wreaking havoc on me and my caregivers.

Who will cure this part of the disease we call *Alzheimer's?*

# "Oh, I've Done That
# Myself a Million Times!"

While lunching with a friend today, I told him of a deep existential fear that is starting to creep into my heart and mind. I am starting to fear the coming of the end of me. Not the *death* of me, but the *end* of me as I know myself and as others have known me. My body will still be around, and like my granddaughter's hermit crab, someone or some thing will crawl inside of me and carry me around for a while until I become too much of a physical burden, and then the crab will leave and my body will stop functioning. It is an interesting question about when I will actually die, but that is another yet unwritten piece.

The consequence of this creeping fear is that I have noticed I have started to pull more into myself. I fear being alone with a stranger whom I don't know, maybe won't like, certainly won't understand as I now know myself, and here I am hastening the process by withdrawing into myself. It seems to be the pattern most people with Alzheimer's follow. Even before we must withdraw because of the failure of our cognitive processes, we begin to pull into ourselves.

The more "errors" I make, the more fearful I am. The more fearful I am of the future, the more I rush into it. In an odd sort of way, it is safer to hide in a dark closet, even if I am afraid of the dark. No one can see me. If I make mistakes reading aloud; if I cannot remember to close the door; if I forget to take out the dog—no one will know. And now I know for sure I have reached a point of self-awareness that I know I don't know. I just don't know when I don't know. I misunderstand what is going on around me. I get confused about the order of occurrences and sometimes draw wrong conclusions based on a mixed up timeline. I don't forget in the sense that when I am cued or reminded it comes to my mind. I have to stop and consider what I have been told I forgot. I have to consider it as if it happened, even though I still have no recollection of it really happening. What if it was the way someone said it was. How would that change what I now feel and believe? But I honestly do not recall it. Have no recollection, at all! Can I successfully live in a world where I am missing larger and larger chunks of what is going on around me?

Now, we all make perceptual errors. We all have our predisposi-
tions, filters, idiosyncrasies, and differences. Yet, we all somehow
manage to reach some agreements that lead to caring and loving

> *Can I successfully
> live in a world where
> I am missing larger
> and larger chunks of
> what is going on
> around me?*

each other, which lead to commitment and
families, which lead to a sense of well being.
I know I am on some occasions *not* okay; I
just don't know when they are happening. I
don't know how to recall and understand
them with the benefit of hindsight. Increasingly, I cannot trust myself to take care of
myself. I know I was never perfect. I know I
could have been better. I know I tried my
best and hardest, most of the time. Now, I
am dealing with the fact that those days are over. I am losing control
of my potential to improve. I am losing control of my ability to
understand myself. These issues of lack of control of myself are leading me to existential fear of losing myself.

Along comes my friend who tells me not to worry because everyone makes mistakes, forgets, and gets confused. I think he called
them *brain farts!* If only they were signs I had consumed beans, instead
of signs that I am moving into another stage of the disease! Others
may see my errors as the same as their own, but to me they are confirmation of what others have been saying for three years: "You have
dementia, probably of the Alzheimer's type."

As Alzheimer's progresses, human beings don't become aliens.
They are still human beings, just repackaged in a way that is unique.
The symptoms and consequences of the disease are not by themselves
unique to this disease. When they come together, whatever the cause
(whatever they eventually will agree causes the disease), the disease
process is labeled as *dementia, of the Alzheimer's type*; it may be true that
separately these are common "human" behaviors that many people
occasionally experience, but this fact is not useful for the person with
the disease.

Well intended as family and friends are—confused and fearful as
they are when they see symptoms in me that can be characterized as
gastric events ("brain farts") in others—they fear losing me and I fear
losing myself. It is not that one fear is greater or more profound than
the other. In fact, I believe as caregivers see the same signs as I (and
they see many more, because I am at a place where I can't see or
understand my mistakes), they too develop an existential fear about

who they are, if they can make it, and will they be successful; and they try harder instead of withdrawing.

So I am withdrawing, those around me are trying harder to engage me, and we cannot appreciate or understand why the other person will not be more like them.

I believe individuals who are confronted by the advancing stages of the disease withdraw prematurely because it is easier, it is safer, and they do not know what else to do. Caregivers who are confronted by the advancing stages of the disease pull harder on us to try to make us feel safer. Ironic, isn't it, that the harder they pull, the more we resist?

We need to engage with each other in a different way. If we haven't yet engaged—you watch me and tell me what *not* to do—then I try but reach a point where I don't know if my trying is or isn't successful—it is very, very difficult to suddenly "connect" with each other. We are scared, we are already trying what we think is best for ourselves and the other person, we are at odds and we know it, but we don't know what to do except keep trying.

Remember, the harder we try to implement our own strategies, the more difficult it becomes for the other people to implement their strategies. This tug-of-war is guaranteed to produce two losers. I will prematurely disappear into myself, and others will prematurely be forced to deal with me in a condition they don't want to happen.

As my grandmother would exclaim, "Oh my!"

# From the Inside Out

# The Chase for Yesterday

In the compulsive gambling community, there is a principle they call "the chase." After a compulsive gambler hits his first really, really big win, he spends the rest of his life chasing after the feeling of that first big score. Unfortunately, as with most addictions, more and more of the addictive substance produces less and less of a high. The person will never, ever feel the high of the first big win. You really cannot go home again!

I am in the early-middle of the Alzheimer's Chase. I am chasing the feeling I had prior to my neurologist saying, "You have Alzheimer's. We do have a medication which seems to slow the progress of the disease in some people, for some time." Unfortunately, the prescribed Alzheimer's medication produced what felt like gallons and gallons of stomach acid. So, naturally, I took another pill to get rid of the stomach acid. My gastroenterologist told me the acid had begun to wear away the lining of my esophagus. "Ultimately," he said, "you might develop throat cancer unless something is done about the acid." Enter yet another proton pump inhibitor, and a pill for the anxiety I felt concerning the possibility of throat cancer. As pills gained control over those side effects, I started to come to grips with the diagnosis of this life-shortening, and dignity-stripping, disease. I became really, really depressed! I took two pills twice a day in an attempt to bring my feelings back to the pre-Alzheimer's days, or at least that was the goal. Oh, and by the way, since I had just turned 60 years old, let's throw in a slightly enlarged prostate and two more pills. Swallowing one and a half handfuls of drugs twice a day offered me the opportunity to become more anxious. How about doubling my anxiety medication? Having trouble with my libido—they have a blue pill for that. Don't forget the OTC (over-the-counter) stuff: vitamin E, vitamin C, vitamin Bs 1-100, fish oil, and a mega pill of multivitamins and minerals.

I am an empty vessel into which I throw a hand and a half full of pills twice a day, and

> *I am an empty vessel into which I throw a hand and a half full of pills twice a day, and I desperately want the pills to reconstruct me.*

I desperately want the pills to reconstruct me into the person I was the day before the chase began—the day before I went to my neurologist.

When will the chase end for me?

What will my costly and all-out efforts to participate in the chase accomplish for me?

Will I ever be "myself" again?

---

Compulsive pathological gambling affects 1%–2% of adults, and up to 4% of adults living within 50 miles of a casino. It is a brain disease that seems to be similar to disorders such as alcoholism and drug addiction. These disorders likely involve problems with the part of the brain associated with behaviors such as eating and sex. This part of the brain is sometimes called the "pleasure center" or dopamine reward pathway.

In people who develop compulsive pathological gambling, occasional gambling leads to habitual gambling. Like alcohol or drug addiction, pathological gambling is a chronic disorder that tends to get worse without treatment. Even with treatment, relapses are common. Nevertheless, people with pathological gambling can do very well with appropriate treatment.

*http://www.nlm.nih.gov/medlineplus/ency/article/001520.htm*

# What's the Up Side to Having Alzheimer's Disease?

*Americans fear getting Alzheimer's disease more than heart disease, stroke, or diabetes.*

—MetLife Foundation Alzheimer's Survey

(http://www.metlife.com/Applications/Corporate/WPS/CDA/PageGenerator/0,4132,P12046,00.html)

Nothing that I can think of, right off the bat, but here are some thoughts on how my life has changed since I was diagnosed with Alzheimer's disease.

I talk more often and longer on the phone with my out-of-town family members.

We talk more about what is going on inside us rather than around us.

We get together more than weddings, funerals, and an occasional Christmas.

I have discovered in my brother and myself a resonance of thought and feeling that I only sensed prior to the diagnosis. My spouse and I have developed a new level and intensity of closeness, an intimacy about our life as husband and wife. One of my children retired early from the Air Force and moved to Houston to help his mother and me. Along with my son and my daughter-in-law came my two grandchildren. Instead of seeing them four times a year, I see them four or more times a day!

I started to write again in my *Simple Abundance Gratitude Journal* (list four things each day for which you feel gratitude and do not repeat them again on your list). I take longer walks with my dog, Annie. We talk more, or at least I do.

I am a better teacher. I care about and try to show it to all my students, even the ones who do not care back. I initiate more e-mail contact, and I promptly answer all who write me. I am planning on a long-postponed rafting trip down the Grand Canyon, and I would like to take a Windjammer cruise (where passengers are a part of the crew on a large schooner).

> *I have learned to recognize the difference between sympathy and empathy, and I have learned how to accept both of them.*

I spend more time feeling and thinking about what is going on inside of me. Sometimes, this is good; most times, it is not. I am more in touch with *me*.

I have learned to recognize the difference between sympathy and empathy, and I have learned how to accept both of them. I don't care as much how well the Chicago Bears are doing this season. Formerly, a loss on their part on Sunday would produce a dour mood in yours truly for most of Monday.

You might say I have a deeper appreciation of what I should and should not respond to emotionally.

I give more of myself and most times expect nothing in return. Is this the "up side," or is this how I should have lived in the first place? In either case, these responses to the disease feel good.

Still, I couldn't really say, as some others with Alzheimer's do, that I am glad that I know that I have Alzheimer's, glad that I got the diagnosis early.

---

If you are a lemonade person rather than a lemon person, consider The Positive Psychology Center. It promotes research, training, education, dissemination, and the application of Positive Psychology.

Positive Psychology seeks to understand and build the strengths and virtues that enable individuals and communities to thrive.

*http://www.ppc.sas.upenn.edu/*

# Pride Precedes the Fall

*The seven deadly sins, also known as the* capital vices *or* cardinal sins, *are a classification of vices used in early Christian teachings to educate and protect followers from basic human instincts. The one that acts as the motivators to seek out the others is Pride.*

—http://en.wikipedia.org/wiki/Seven_deadly_sins

I have never thought of myself as a vain person, but I am prideful. I feel pride about the way I do things. I feel pride in my ability to accomplish things.

For the past 22 years, I have been making liqueurs for my family and friends at Christmas. I personalize the labels with the recipient's name. This year was to be no different. I cannot remember the multiple times both my wife and son asked me if I needed any help. "Of course not," I claimed. "I have been making these for 22 years."

I forgot to include the vanilla in my amaretto and made two spelling mistakes on the labels I printed. I was not aware of these mistakes, and others, until after I had mailed all the bottles. I mixed up bottles and mailing addresses. Some people received someone else's bottle. I made one batch of amaretto at half strength. And, those are only the mistakes of which I am aware!

I have always taken pride in what I do. I am no perfectionist—ask my spouse, who is one! I enjoy the process of doing things, and most of my feelings of accomplishment come from the middle, not the end, of projects. I care about how things turn out, but I take pride in the way I did them.

> *I enjoy the process of doing things, and most of my feelings of accomplishment come from the middle, not the end, of projects.*

I have reached the point in the disease process where I make a lot of "mistakes." I am immediately aware of some mistakes. Some mistakes others make me aware of, and I suspect there are many mistakes of which I am simply unaware. I feel very bad about this situation. I cannot always control how I perform the process; therefore, I cannot produce the feeling of pride in a process well done.

In fact, I am not in control of some of my own behaviors.

Why don't I ask for help?

Why don't I seek out help?

Why don't I let others help me to avoid the mistakes I know I am going to make?

My own sense of pride keeps me from accepting the help of others, especially for simple tasks. It is humiliating to ask for help with tasks, such as making liqueurs, that I have been doing for the past 22 years! However, the fact is at this stage of the disease, my quest for self-worth has become counterproductive. In addition to the disease, I am becoming my own enemy!

Pride, coupled with Alzheimer's, creates a "deadly sin." I am falling and losing my pride, both at the same time. Pride may hasten my fall!

One can never *truly* stand in another's shoes. However, when others without Alzheimer's disease try their best to stand in our shoes, to experience the world as people with Alzheimer's do, it helps both of us.

---

*Pride* (vanity, narcissism)

A desire to be more important or attractive to others, failing to give credit due to others, or excessive love of self (especially holding self out of proper position toward God). Dante's definition was "love of self perverted to hatred and contempt for one's neighbor." Pride was what sparked the fall of Lucifer from Heaven. The absolute of the three exaggerated adulthood sins, as a prideful person believes him/herself to be in complete control of things. The seven deadly sins are Pride, Envy, Wrath, Sloth, Greed, Gluttony, and Lust.

*http://en.wikipedia.org/wiki/Seven_deadly_sins*

# HOW MANY PEOPLE HAVE DEMENTIA?

The world's population is aging. Currently, there are an estimated 24 million people world-wide with dementia. Two thirds of these live in developing countries. This figure is set to increase to more than 80 million people by 2040. Much of this increase will be in rapidly developing and heavily populated regions such as China, India, and Latin America.

Dementia primarily affects older people. Up to the age of 65, dementia develops in only about 1 person in 1,000. The chance of having the condition rises sharply with age to 1 person in 20 over the age of 65. Over the age of 80, this figure increases to 1 person in 5.

*http://www.alz.co.uk/alzheimers/faq.html#howmany*

# Safe and Sound . . .
# Unsound and Safe

While walking in the mall last week, I saw a table set up by our local police department at which they offered to fingerprint and videotape children for identification purposes. Children as old as 12 years of age were uncomfortably standing in line. Like diamond rings, automobiles, and my grandmother's silver, we now register and photograph our children in case they are stolen or become lost.

Yesterday, I asked my four-year-old granddaughter to help me fasten my Safe Return bracelet around my arm. I had been thinking of doing this for several months. I asked my granddaughter to help me because I didn't want to make a big deal of this with caregivers and, perhaps more important, with myself.

Occasionally, I get lost. I go to places I didn't intend to go. I have moments, especially in strange places, when my confusion shifts into bewilderment and I am for the briefest of moments not sure what is going on around me. It is very difficult for me to accept the idea that I would ever need Safe Return, most especially now or tomorrow, or tomorrow's tomorrow.

I don't feel like a diamond ring or an automobile or even a tarnished piece of my grandmother's silver, but I think I know the confusion and fear that children must feel when being fingerprinted and videotaped. "Those upon whom I sometimes depend to take care of me are admitting that sometimes even they can't take care of me. I can't be trusted to take care of myself. The world is an unfriendly place to those of us who can't always take care of ourselves. People might not always remember what I look like, so they will make a video. People want to know it is me, for sure, even when they can't recognize me, so they take my fingerprints."

*Am I reassured Safe Return will protect me, or am I reminded daily of my impending inability to know where and who I am?*

Is this reassuring, or does it feed insecurities and fears? Am I reassured Safe Return will protect me, or am I reminded daily of my impending in-ability to know where and who I am?

I am telling and showing the world I can't always trust myself to know myself. I am wearing a billboard asking for help, even when I might not want or need to ask. I am always telling others some-thing about me. I'm not sure it is any of their business knowing, un-less I want to tell them. It's okay for family to know. It's okay for those I choose to tell to know. But the whole world? I'm not sure.

I am constantly aware I am wearing the Safe Return bracelet. I thought after a week or two I would get used to it, like wearing a ring. I suppose I will always be aware of it until I am not aware.

---

The single best piece of advice I can offer to anyone involved with one of the diseases of de-mentia is to register with Safe Return—a nationwide identification system designed to assist in the safe return of people who become lost when wandering. Contact your local Alzheim-er's Association for details.

# I Am a Verb

*VERB*
*Function: noun (Isn't it ironic, confusing, and*
*interesting that the word* verb *is a noun?)*
*Meaning: A word that denotes an action or a state*
—Web Dictionary, 2006

Frustrated with General McClellan's reactive strategy to win the Civil War, President Abraham Lincoln interviewed Ulysses Simpson Grant for the position as General Commander of the Union Army. Lincoln saw Grant as a man of action, a proactive strategist. Grant, so the story goes in his autobiography, was asked by Lincoln to describe himself in one one word. Grant responded, "I am a verb." He thought of himself as a verb, a general who was a doer. Living and fighting in a world of nouns, Grant was a man of action. After a bloody defeat, there was a call for him to be fired. Lincoln replied, "I can't fire him. He is a general who fights." He was a verb who knew how to keep nouns in their place.

I, on the other hand, was a personal pronoun. I was a person, place, or thing. After 61 years, lots of people knew me as the pronoun *Richard Taylor.* I was a consistent, caring, and comfortable pronoun. Gregarious and outspoken, as I was, people had a good idea of how I thought and in what I believed. I was, dare I say, predictable. I offered no surprises when I opened my mouth. My way was the best way, until someone convinced me otherwise. It took a strong verb to get me to change my mind! I pretty much ignored the nouns around me and did what I thought needed to be done, not what the nouns or, for that matter, the verbs said should be done. I was a strong pronoun, seldom influenced by annoying verbs. When I said I would do something, I did it. When I thought I understood a problem, I solved it. I was consistent, straightforward, and dependable.

I, too, am a verb. I am still a man of action, but I change from time to time, depending on my tense. I morph, depending on my morphemes (*s, ed, ing, en*). Tense, aspect, voice, modality, and most especially mood are now major influences on who I am and how I act. I am a man of unpredictable actions, inappropriate actions. My actions reveal a confused and sometimes bewildered verb who is not quite sure if, when, where, and how he should react to the nouns who surround him. Richard Taylor, the pronoun, is now Richard Taylor/Alzheimer's disease. I am a verb—I be, I do. Exactly what "I be" and how "I do" depends on my disease. Who I will be tomorrow is anyone's guess. In fact, who I will be tonight or in an hour or in the next five minutes is anyone's

> *When I said I would do something, I did it. When I thought I understood a problem, I solved it. I was a leader who was consistent, straightforward, and dependable.*

guess. I join Ulysses in being an unpredictable entity—good for a general who wants to keep his opponent off guard, but bad for a human being who wants to be trusted, loved, and perceived as dependable.

Since the diagnosis and my subsequent "retirement," I have a lot more time available to me. I am learning lots of new nouns: amyloid, tau, endoplasmic reticulum, person-centered caregiving, and pain management. I am surrounded by nouns that seem to be acting on me rather than me acting on them. How I direct these nouns to act changes from doctor's visit to doctor's visit. It depends on how I feel and what I can remember. There is no guarantee that I will act the same way twice. When I say I will do something, sometimes I will and sometimes I won't. I forget. I make lists to remember other lists and then sometimes forget both sets of lists. When I think I understand a problem, someone points out that I have neglected to consider some facts which I forgot to consider or do not remember ever

knowing in the first place. I am now consistently inconsistent. I still remain straightforward, but who I am and how I am thinking keeps changing, sometimes from day to day or hour to hour. You can depend on me to be undependable, but that is about all you can depend on.

> *I still remain straightforward, but who I am and how I am thinking keeps changing, sometimes from day to day or hour to hour.*

I am now relentlessly inconsistent. As the verb changes, so does the noun. There is no longer the security of knowing that I am the same yesterday, today, and tomorrow.

When I act out or act uncharacteristically, caregivers charitably attribute the actions to the verb, not the noun. "It's the disease, not Richard." Grammatically there may be a difference, but in the real world, they are now one and the same. I am Alzheimer's, and Alzheimer's is me. I struggled to remain a pronoun as the ever-changing verb struggles to change me. The verb is increasingly in control and winning. All diseases, but especially those like Alzheimer's that live between our ears, cause us to act as verbs. The diseases change us as they progress, producing more and different symptoms.

As Grant lay in his bed, dying from throat cancer, according to one of his chroniclers his last recorded words were "I am a verb." I shall die, probably being unable to say anything. But those around me will know that at that moment, "I am Alzheimer's disease"—the disease that turned me from a pronoun to a verb.

---

Born Hiram Ulysses Grant in Point Pleasant, Clermont County, Ohio. At the age of 17, having barely passed the United States Military Academy's height requirement for entrance, Grant received a nomination to the Academy at West Point. His congressman mistakenly nominated him as Ulysses Simpson Grant, knowing Grant's mother's maiden name and forgetting that Grant was referred to in his youth as "H. Ulysses Grant" or "Lyss." Grant wrote his name in the entrance register as "Ulysses Hiram Grant" (concerned that he would otherwise become known by his initials, H.U.G.), but the school administration refused to accept any name other than the nominated form.

My full name is Richard Ralph Taylor (RRT). I did have an uncle who called me "Rail Road Track"!

*http://en.wikipedia.org/wiki/Ulysses_S._Grant*

# Whatever Happened to Hope?

Google the word *hope* and it responds with 1,100,000,000 web pages that contain the word *hope*. Hope seems pretty important, at least among web page developers. (There are only 746,000,000 hits for the word *sex!*). I was always a hopeful person. I was always hoping for something that wasn't there: world peace, no cavities, a *Father Knows Best* family, a thicker lawn, a more forgiving me, more money, a bigger and longer automobile, et cetera and so forth. I know lots of people who are hoping their lives will improve when: the kids move out, they get married, they get divorced, they are promoted, the brown spot in their lawn does not return next year, they finally retire, or they reach a "better place" after they die.

Since I was diagnosed with Alzheimer's disease, I no longer hope.

I gave up hoping when I found out that hope was never going to reverse the quickening death of my brain cells and my hastened death. I gave up hoping when I realized that hoping by itself creates disappointment, because what you hoped for never happens exactly the way you hoped it would. Only Jimmy Stewart had all his hopes fully realized. Wasn't that a movie?

I abandoned hope when I realized how much of my attention and energy, which was invested in continually hoping for a better tomorrow, drained my focus from today. Hope does not keep me alive; it ensures I will never be happy today because I am hoping things will be better tomorrow.

Since all I have for sure and all I know for sure is today, why should I invest time and energy today in hoping things will be better tomorrow, or next week, or in a year?

Hope helped me avoid responsibility for making the most of today. I spent time hoping that tomorrow would be better than today. Hope was the reason I didn't make the most of today. Hope acted as a substitute for action today, because I hoped some one or some thing would make tomorrow better,

> *The fact that I know I have Alzheimer's disease motivates my focus on actively making today better than yesterday, not hoping tomorrow will be better than today.*

and my own actions today would not be necessary to make tomorrow better.

Some people, although not I, have faith that tomorrow may be better because some higher power has intervened in the affairs of men and women and cured their loved one of Alzheimer's disease. They hope that, based on their faith, a higher power will listen and then act on their specific request. They miss part of the joy of today while hoping tomorrow will be more joyful.

The fact that I know I have Alzheimer's disease motivates my focus on actively making today better than yesterday, not hoping tomorrow will be better than today.

*Carpe diem!* (Seize the day!!)

---

My opinions concerning the role hope plays in my life have consistently generated strong responses from readers both for and against my beliefs. Here are some other perspectives on hope.

*Hope* may be emotional belief in the possibility of positive outcomes related to events and circumstances within your personal life. It implies a certain amount of perseverance. Hope may be different than:

*Faith:* Hope is subordinate to faith in that while hope is emotional, faith carries a divinely inspired and informed form of positive belief. Hope is typically contrasted with despair, which connotes an ignorance of religious faith; hope likewise carries a connotation of being informed.

*Optimism:* Whereas optimism refers to a positive view at a conceptual or intellectual level, hope refers to a positive belief at the emotional level. Optimism may be rational and informed by facts; hope may lack a strong connection to reality.

*Positive thinking:* Hope is distinct from positive thinking, a therapeutic or systematic process used in psychology for reversing pessimism.

*http://en.wikipedia.org/wiki/Hope*

# *Moving from Living with My Mind to Living in My Mind*

✕✦✕✦✕✦✕✦✕

Currently I am of two minds. Ever since I was diagnosed with Alzheimer's disease, my mind has taken on a life, a form, and even an imagined personality of its own. I am, at least in my mind, a person of and with two minds. This dualism within my mind, by my mind, is what allows me to still maintain some personal sense of who I am, who I was, and who I am becoming. My Alzheimer's diseased mind is something I think about. It is something I can picture in the rest of my "other" mind. It has good days and bad days. It has a disease that is slowly killing it.

I know it is not healthy to live with more than one voice or person inside of you, but I have managed to push my diseased mind into a corner and, to some extent, separate myself from it. I live with the disease, but the disease lives in my mind, not in me. I can observe it. I can speak about it, think about it, and worry about it. Thus far, it has not spoken back, thank heavens! Soon there will be a meeting of the minds, and ominously, with each passing day, they become one and the same mind. I am being absorbed into my diseased mind. Eventually, I will be one diseased mind, living in that mind and not in the world as I now know it.

> *Right now I am more concerned with the transition, the process, the journey, from being of two minds to being of one diseased mind.*

Right now I am more concerned with the transition, the process, the journey, from being of two minds to being of one diseased mind. I understand that I have no influence or control over where I will end up. It's the thought of jumping back and forth from my diseased mind to myself and back in again that frightens me. It's talking with people in the second and third stages of the disease and hearing and watching them struggle with the jolt of moving back and forth that frightens me. It is hearing and watching caregivers struggle with the jolt of their loved ones moving from living with their minds to living in their diseased minds that saddens me.

Why can't my mind just make up its mind? Why must I spend years intermittently knowing and being who I was, and then plunging back into who I have become? Sometimes knowledge is not power, it is a curse!

---

There are three broad stages to Alzheimer's. In the beginning, the patient may notice his or her own forgetfulness and will solicit others' help or write lists. In the second phase there will be severe memory loss, particularly for recent events. A sufferer may often remember long-ago events while being unable to remember a just-viewed TV show. In this stage, disorientation usually begins, dysphasia (inability to find the right word) may occur, and mood changes happen that can be unpredictable and sudden. By the third stage, people with Alzheimer's experience severe confusion and disorientation, and may suffer hallucinations or delusions. Some may become violent or angry, while others may be docile or helpless. In this stage, sufferers may wander without purpose, experience incontinence, and neglect personal hygiene.

*http://www.fda.gov/fdac/features/1998/398_alz.html*

# And the Name of the 3,000-Pound Elephant Is "Fear"

X◆X◆X◆X◆X

*I fear I am not in my perfect mind.*
*Methinks I should know you and know this man;*
*Yet, I am doubtful; for I am mainly ignorant*
*What place this is; and all the skill I have*
*Remembers not these garments; nor I know not*
*Where I did lodge last night. Do not laugh at me.*
—William Shakespeare, *King Lear* (IV, 7)

It is 4 A.M., and in an effort to distract my mind from continuing a horrible nightmare, I have stumbled across what is for me one of the secrets deeply buried under ounces of brain cell bunkers of Dr. Alzheimer. I have been struggling for months in therapy to discover my own primal, explosive, and contaminating Alzheimer's issues. For me, issues are like tumors that have been growing inside of me since first my mother refused to pick me up when I was hungry. Did she really love me? Would she ever have time for me, to meet my needs? Where was Dad when I needed him? (You fans of psychoanalysis know the rest of the psychobabble.)

Along comes Alzheimer's disease, and the mind begins to grow yet another set of tumors, which actually arise and are dependent on the original set of tumors. These Alzheimer tumors grow much faster than the primal tumors, quickly reaching the surface of my personality.

These tumors don't need blood to grow. They are fed by copious amounts of fear, a leftover of evolution in all of us from our fight/flight response as subhumans. The announcement of the diagnosis includes a huge injection of fear, hitherto unknown by the recipient. The secure become fearful. The fearful feel overwhelmed. The overwhelmed feel as if they can't make it.

My two largest and most active tumors, fed by my fear that was activated when Dr. Hennan accidentally stuck me in the eye with his thumb as I was entering the world (just kidding), are my growing sense of my loss of independence and my growing dependence on others. These fears come as a matched set!

I cannot drive; therefore, I must depend on others to take me everywhere. I cannot cook; therefore, I must depend on someone to cook for me. I cannot take care of my money; therefore, I must depend on someone else to manage my finances. I cannot trust myself to remember the simplest of ideas; therefore, I must depend on others to tell me where to go, what to do, and when to do it. The paired list goes on and on.

I believe that at some point in time, relatively soon, these parallel tumors will meet and become one giant tumor. At that moment, the tumor will no longer be a concern of mine. I will fear no more. When my mind has reached this level of malignancy, new fears even more powerful than my previous fears will emerge from an as yet undiscovered bunker and I will live in a new world, wrestling with fears which no one who does not already live there can comprehend. I will be someone or something other than I am right now.

Even assuming my best efforts and the efforts of one of the best therapists in my community, I do not believe I have enough time or brain power to conquer these fears. I grow less independent and more dependent with each sunrise and sunset. My best, and perhaps only, strategy and hope is to avoid the consequences of my growing fears—consequences I believe are captured by the word *depression!* Every morning, I stand up to the fears and say to myself, "So what? I can't be scared, unless I choose to scare myself." Daily, I say to myself, "What's the big deal? So what if you are losing some of your independence and are swallowing more dependence? You thought you were going to be the first human being not to grow old? You thought you would live forever? Get real, Richard. You have enough problems with your body without creating more thorny intellectual constructs in your mind!"

"Yes, but what about fear, fear of death, fear of being out of control, fear of what I am doing to my caregivers' lives, fear of loss of dignity, fear of the loss of self, fear of the unknown, fear of fear—the list of fears I have could fill a 1-gig hard disk."

I know my fears are irrational. I know that fear, as I am experiencing it now, is irrational. A tad here and there is good for babies and adolescents. It helps keep "moral" people moral. It protects us from making inappropriate and unhealthy decisions.

Most likely I will be unaware of the moment when I am completely dependent on others and have lost my own independence. As I have grown older, I have become aware that I am already stumbling down both of these roads. Alzheimer's disease has made steeper the grade of both of these roads. What began as a stroll has now evolved into a trot, to be followed by an all-out run, and culminating in an out-of-control tumble to where the bottomless pit of helplessness awaits me. Is it rational to believe that I alone would maintain the level of independence I attained when I moved out of my parents' house? When I got my first job? Is it rational to believe that I alone would maintain the level of control obtained when I reached the peak of my earnings? When I finally discovered and loved myself?

Unlike the tumors of my lifelong issues, Alzheimer's tumors are impervious to rational or logical attacks. In many cases, it is physically impossible for an individual with Alzheimer's disease to use logic and evidence as the basis for attacking and overcoming irrational beliefs. In therapy, I discovered the irrational basis of my fears. I identified many of my counterproductive and self-destructive behaviors. I then opened the door of my therapist's office and proceeded to repeat the fear-driven behaviors over and over again. While this is a practice common to many people without Alzheimer's (changing human behavior is not as easy as Albert Ellis makes it out to be), they always have the possibility of changing from within. I am losing that possibility. I can feel my free will slipping away. My ability to observe myself and change myself as a result of my observations is not what it used to be. Sometimes, many times, I am not only unaware I am doing something, I can't recall having done it. These growing mental blind spots are serious impediments to a rational approach to living! In the past, memory, thoughts, and insight were my tools for analysis and change. Now I am working with unsure memory, sometimes bizarre thoughts (can everyone be against me?), and insights which are fewer in number and which I trust less and less.

> *In many cases, it is physically impossible for an individual with Alzheimer's disease to use logic and evidence as the basis for attacking and overcoming irrational beliefs.*

I believe everyone lives with fear feeding the tumors of their personalities. What differentiates individuals experiencing atypical physical changes in their brains and the rest of the population is our ability to use our rational-thinking toolchest of defensive weapons against our fears. If individuals with Alzheimer's attempt to ignore the fertilizing effects of fear on their personalities, they open themselves to the real risk of being overwhelmed by their fears!

The double whammy of thinking about my loss of independence and my increasing dependence has led me to the point where I understand more clearly that this is not a universal truth for everyone growing old. Specifically, for me, someone with Alzheimer's disease, fear is the 3,000-pound elephant tromping around in my mind. If I ignore it and pretend it isn't there, I do so at my own risk. I have never learned how to train this elephant. Now that it has suddenly grown 1,000-fold, I fear it is out of control and frankly beyond control! I fear the consequences. I fear the consequences for my caregivers!

(Aren't mixed metaphors interesting and challenging to understand in their totality?)

Fear is an unpleasant feeling of perceived risk or danger, whether it be real or imagined. Fear also can be described as a feeling of extreme dislike toward certain conditions, objects, people, or situations (e.g., fear of darkness, ghosts). It is one of the basic emotions and is linked heavily to the amygdala neurons.

Fear may underlie some alterations in expected behaviors.

Fear inside a person has different degrees and varies from one person to another. If not properly handled, fear can lead to social problems and health problems.

Some philosophers have considered fear to be a useless emotion; other thinkers note the usefulness of fear as a warning of potentially unpleasant situations or consequences. Still others consider that fear is the fuel that feeds the ego's (as in "separating/judgmental agent") engine.

*http://en.wikipedia.org/wiki/Fear*

# It's On the Tip of My Tongue

All of us have had the experience of sensing that we know what the right word is, but we can't quite access it. In fact, we say, "It's on the tip of my tongue." This tip of the tongue phenomenon (TOTP) has been studied by psychologists, linguists, and others interested in finding external clues concerning the internal processes of our brains. We actually have a sense that some process is running in our brain but we can't access it. We must let it run its course until it releases its product to be spoken by the tongue.

Some time not too long ago, I must have bitten off the tip of my tongue and not realized what happened. I went through a period during which I thought if I would just relax and not panic, the thought for which I was searching would form itself and sort of bubble up into my consciousness. I had to learn to just trust myself.

Imagine living in my world where now I can no longer trust myself, my tongue, and my mind to access, form, and bubble up into my consciousness the word or thought I am seeking. I'm not talking about polysyllabic words. I'm looking for my granddaughter's name. I'm waiting for the name of the professional football team I've been following for 40 years to bubble up into my conscious mind. I need to find and say my home address, my phone number, the date of my own birth!

> *I'm not talking about polysyllabic words. I'm looking for my granddaughter's name.*

These days, I'm moving from searching for the right word to searching for the thought! Increasingly, it is not a matter of waiting for the correct noun, verb, adverb, or adjective to pop up and out. It is a matter of waiting to discover an entire fact. Did I drive my car here? Did I already read this? Did I even bring my keys? I yearn for the TOTP—the feeling of knowing it is there but it just hasn't come out yet. I don't know if it's there or not. I do know that it probably won't come out. I can no longer trust that it will!

# IMPORTANCE OF MEMORY SCREENINGS

- Memory screenings are a first step toward finding out if you have Alzheimer's disease or a related dementia, or another type of condition that is causing memory loss.

- A memory screening is not used to diagnose any particular illness. A screening can test your memory, language skills, thinking ability, and other intellectual functions. It can indicate whether you might benefit from more testing. If the screening raises concern, see your doctor or other health care professional and get a complete examination.

- Memory can be affected by a number of factors, ranging from stress and lack of sleep, to illnesses such as Alzheimer's disease and vascular dementia.

- Early recognition of mild cognitive impairment (MCI)—mild intellectual loss that may develop into dementia—provides an opportunity for health care professionals to treat this condition and possibly slow the decline in memory and other functions.

- For irreversible illnesses, such as Alzheimer's disease, early diagnosis could improve your future health. Although there currently is no cure for Alzheimer's disease, available and emerging medical treatments may slow the progression of symptoms. These medications have been proven to work best the earlier they are given.

- Early diagnosis can improve quality of life. Individuals can learn more about the disease, get counseling and other social services support, address legal and financial issues, and have more of a say about their care.

*http://www.nationalmemoryscreening.org*

# "I Can Read!"
# "I Can't."

I am working with my five-year-old granddaughter to teach her how to read. She knows the alphabet, each of the letter sounds, some phonetic combinations, and some words. The other day, I was reading a book to her at naptime and we came across a sentence that she could read in its entirety. She interrupted me, read the sentence, and announced to me with a broad grin on her face (and a tear in my right eye), "I can read, Grandpa. I can read!"

Later that same day, I was reading her a story at bed time, stumbling over the words, ignoring some of them, repeating myself, and saying some sentences that just didn't make sense. She turned to me and said, "Grandpa, did you forget how to read?"

Two years ago, while I was a member of a support group with other individuals with Alzheimer's, the therapist asked, "How many of you cannot read?" About half the group raised their hands. I remember thinking, "How can you forget to read? What must life be like if you can't read? Why aren't they more upset that they can't read?"

I now know the answers to my own questions. It isn't that I can't read. I understand words, and grammar, and how to read. I know how to read! I just can't. Rather than deal with the hassle of reading simple newspaper articles over and over again to fully understand the news, I have started to skim the headlines. After all, I can't recall much of what I read (originally, a tragedy of major proportions for me), so why should I waste my time reading for understanding of the details? I can still read street signs, instructions, and so forth. Saying "I can't read" is inaccurate. I can't fully comprehend. I can't always understand everything. I mispronounce, misunderstand, and ignore words when reading—especially aloud. Thank heavens for voice recognition software. It has helped me make this book possible.

> It isn't that I can't read. I understand words, and grammar, and how to read. I know how to read! I just can't.

It has probably extended my ability to communicate through e-mail by at least a year!

For reasons I cannot imagine, I still talk okay! The members of my group all talked okay, even those who raised their hands. I have started to notice that I sometimes type the same initial four or five words of a sentence two times, sort of like I am stuttering. Occasionally, a stray word will pop up in a sentence of my e-mail. Whoever invented spell checkers and grammar checkers . . . a thousand alms upon your body! I write more and more using a voice-to-computer dictation program. I spend lots and lots of time going over and over my transcripts to edit them to make sense to me and to others.

My granddaughter and I are switching from me reading to listening to tapes of someone else reading while we look at the book. She actually likes it better because the "different voices" are better than mine. There are music and sound effects I can't hope to replicate. We listen, look at the pictures, and comment on the story and the pictures. I'm not sure this is going to help her read, but she finds it much more entertaining and interesting, and, frankly, so do I.

But, I still can't read, even if I can . . . if you get what I mean.

# Sing-a-long with Alois and Richard

I was watching TV last night and I stumbled across a rerun of a rerun of a rerun of an old, old, old Billy Graham rally from somewhere in the world where only he and George Beverly Shea spoke English. As the rally ended and he called the multitude to come forward, the massed chorus started to sing, "Just as I am without one plea. . . ." using words I could not pronounce. Halfway through the first verse I found myself singing along (in English, of course). By the second verse, I was shouting along. As they awkwardly transitioned into "What a Friend We Have in Jesus," I awkwardly transitioned right along with them. In fact, we all sang along for another 10 minutes until Cliff Barrows hushed us with a commercial for the Billy Graham Evangelical Association.

I did not rush to the TV and place my hands on its face, nor did I rush to my checkbook and write out a check in the amount I thought would keep me in good standing with God for the next couple of months. (I was raised as a Lutheran, migrated to Unitarianism, and now my religious affiliation and beliefs seem to defy conventional organized religion.)

I was not converted.

I was uplifted!

Alzheimer's is eating my memory, twisting my executive functions, and getting me lost more times than I can count. All of this is wearing on my spirit, but the disease itself cannot consume it. I must do that myself.

Singing something, anything, from children's songs to hymns, from the Hallelujah Chorus from Handel's Messiah (I can still recall the first note for tenors) to any and all Beatles songs, helps me feel that I am feeling okay and, in fact, good.

Humming is also good. It makes your lips, mouth, and throat feel good, in addition to stimulating you to feel good between your ears and in your heart.

It is best to sing out loud and loudly. Thinking about singing is like thinking about sex. It is much, much more satisfying if done with all of your body instead of just between your ears. It is much, much more satisfying if others can and do join in.

I am also a firm supporter of listening to music through a good pair of headphones. If you can't sing, at least listen. Better yet, listen and then sing out of tune! My preference is classical music, opera, and country and western. I am open-minded enough to appreciate that other schools of music can have the same impact on others as these do on me.

*Singing something, anything, from children's songs to hymns . . . helps me feel that I am feeling okay and, in fact, good.*

Not only will words by themselves never hurt you, if sung out loud they can stimulate memories, feelings, and your soul in ways that reading or listening can never come close to. In fact, you don't even have to know the words: "Blah, Blah, Blah," if sung close to the tune, will suffice. Try to know most of the tune. (If you don't know the second verse, just sing the first verse again. No one will notice!) It's even better if you can harmonize or think you can harmonize. I spend a lot of time researching, thinking about, and responding to the sticks and stones of Alzheimer's disease. It is my learned way of dealing with my fears and my situation. Eventually, the disease will break enough of my bones and I will die.

Only I can break my spirit.

I am going to do more singing. I feel safe, sound, healthy, and alive when I sing!

This is my favorite piece of my writing. For some reason, I keep going back to this and rereading it. It makes me feel good inside. (R.T.)

# My Shirt Is Broken

At some moment in the Neolithic Age (6,800–3,300 B.C.), someone tired of his loin cloth constantly falling off and exposing sensitive parts of his/her body to wind, rain, cold, sun, and the eyes of others. He (or she) picked up a piece of bone from the ground, tore two small holes at either side of the loin cloth, inserted the bone, and invented the button.

Women who were members of the upper class of Roman society were restricted to wearing the same type of outer garments as were slave women. They tried to distinguish themselves with fancy hair arrangements. One day, some woman, whose name is lost to history, decided to fasten the sleeve of her outer garment with a piece of bone she had decorated. The button was reinvented!

After diapers and pins (I was invented before Velcro), I discovered the button. I have been buttoning up and down my shirts for more than 60 years. Lately, buttons are again falling out of fashion. Few men get dressed up anymore. First it was zippers, then it was Velcro, then it was t-shirts, and now it is the informal professional look. All of these inventions and trends have contributed to the contemporary death of the button.

Since I retired (a euphemism for "I was forced to quit teaching before I wanted to because of the impact of the disease on my memory and executive abilities"), I don't have many occasions that require me to button up my dress shirt. It is not that I now wander around in the nude or in my bathrobe, but seldom does the occasion present itself when I feel compelled to wear something that buttons up. When a buttoned-shirt occasion does arise, there next to me stands Dr. Alzheimer.

We are going out to a "nice" restaurant with my son and his family. This in my mind requires that I wear a shirt that buttons up the front, instead of a T-shirt. (Although when I arrived there were many T-shirts, lots of baseball hats, two shirts that I can only catalog as colored undershirts, and one guy with a very skimpy shirt, but he had a lot of tattoos.)

But back to my shirt. As I stand here looking in our bathroom mirror and putting on my shirt, I remind myself that I sometimes have difficulty matching up the buttons and the button holes in such a way that when I reach the bottom of the shirt, there are no button holes or buttons left. I make a mental note to check this as I begin to button my shirt from the top down. By the time I reach the bottom of my shirt, I'm attempting to remember the name of the restaurant to which we are going so I can decide before we arrive what it is I want to eat. Now I'm brushing my teeth as my spouse says to me, "Honey, check the buttons on your shirt." I inspect each one of the buttons on my shirt and find each one of them to be in good condition.

Now I'm brushing my hair as my spouse says to me, "Honey, did you check the buttons on your shirt?" I glance at the buttons on my shirt, as reflected in my mirror, and they all look okay to me. As I look down at my shirt, I notice it is unusually uneven at the bottom of the shirt. I did it again, I incorrectly buttoned my shirt! I unbutton the entire shirt and begin to rebutton it, this time with the full attention of my executive functions and mustering all the resources left in my hippocampus. I am determined to get it right

> *I inspect each one of the buttons on my shirt and find each one of them to be in good condition.*

this time. As I somewhat impatiently reach the bottom button, I glance in the mirror for one last check and notice the need for a tad more gel on the left side of my head, just above my ear. That particular cowlick has given me trouble since I was six years old! As we head out the door, I am greeted by my granddaughter, who says, "Grandpa, you buttoned your shirt wrong!"

Without hesitation, I confidently reply, "My shirt is broken."

Even without thinking, I am defensive. Without malice or forethought, I'm covering up my perceived shortcomings. My shirt isn't broken; it is I who am broken. Or am I really broken, or just wrestling with a deteriorating mental condition? In any case, I still don't seem to want anyone to know, perhaps including even myself! Or, am I just a funny grandfather?

The button is interesting. It has a history, an evolution. It began as a simple on/off device and has become a central part of our human culture. We reach out to manipulate objects. We push buttons and magic things happen.

At first, the light goes on. The light goes off. But now, we find our friends and family. We order and ship presents. We launch bombs. The button is the center of our power.

*http://www.louisrosenfeld.com/home/bloug_archive/000455.html*

# Am I Half Empty or Half Full?

A m I becoming something or someone that I wasn't, or am I losing something that I was and will no longer be? Is my life filled with new opportunities for growth, happiness, and enjoyment, or has my life been emptied of opportunities as I sadly shrink into someone nobody knows, including myself?

On good days, I am halfway convinced that the diagnosis of Alzheimer's disease has provided for me the opportunities to become closer to my family, to appreciate today more, and to relish the joys in the hitherto unnoticed details of life. On other days, I am halfway convinced the diagnosis of Alzheimer's disease is slowly emptying my life of closeness, joy, and an appreciation of the details of life. So, am I half full or half empty? The optimists of the world say as long as there is the possibility of self-actualization in your life, and between your ears, you should seek it out. Death, pain, and unhappiness are the means to better focus ourselves on the joy of living. The pessimists of the world say it's a slippery slope, and once the diagnosis has been made, the best you can do is slow down the inevitable plunge into the dark arms of death. And, by the way, you will pay an additional price for slowing down the plunge. You will experience more pain and disappointment for a longer period of time than had you simply let go in the first place.

I don't know why, but people are always asking me if I see myself as half empty or half full. I haven't come up with a satisfying answer—an answer that either they or I will except. Perhaps it is the wrong question. Perhaps it is looking at life from too simplistic a view.

Does a fish know if it is half empty or half full? Do whales ponder their condition and belch to themselves, "Are we half empty or half full?" What about the dolphins swimming around the pool at Sea World, jumping through hoops to receive a fish or two? Do they return to their cages and squeal about their plight in terms of half empty or half full?

Humans are blessed with relatively giant frontal lobes in their brains which allows them to step beyond "am I hungry or not" and think about how hungry they are. Are they hungry enough to appear on reality TV and eat slugs and cockroaches? How unhappy are they?

Unhappy enough to see no future and therefore end their lives? Unhappy enough to pay a therapist a co-pay and talk about their future?

Finally, after 62 years of living, I am beginning to see the gray in life's experience as the heart of the experience. I am not disappointed that it wasn't the best or the worst. I am not judging each experience against another, or against what someone on the TV told me to use as the standard. I am beginning to appreciate the shades of gray. I no longer measure life's experiences against going to the dentist for the first time versus my first sexual experience. A lot of interesting stuff has happened to me along that continuum. In fact, the most valuable experiences for me do not fall on that continuum. They hover above it in a vague, ill-defined cloud, which is always changing shape.

I appreciate and sometimes immerse myself in the process rather than only or mostly on the outcome. I like doing things. I like and appreciate the doing. Doing is how I know I am alive, and how I appreciate being alive.

The more I have observed myself and thought about my experiences since my diagnosis, the more I have discovered how poisoned my life is by, of all people, Aristotle. You know, of course, he was a biologist by trade. And, as such, his goal was to catalog everything. If it was a fish or a reptile, an inductive or deductive argument, or right or wrong, Aristotle had a box to put it in. The more enlightened you were, the more boxes you had. The smarter you were, the better able you were to merge your piles of boxes into fewer and fewer piles.

Living is not about catalogs, boxes, good and evil, right or wrong. Living is about experience, feelings, perspective, and growth.

It is right to kill thousands of people you do not know, but hate, in a declared or undeclared war. It is wrong to kill one person you do not know or hate because you want food for your baby or dope for your soul. You should love your neighbor as yourself, but I have honestly yet to meet one person who loves themselves in a way that should be the template for love for the entire world.

> *Living is not about catalogs, boxes, good and evil, right or wrong. Living is about experience, feelings, perspective, and growth.*

There are lots of "how to" books about how to live, but when you carefully study the lives of the writers you have to wonder why they didn't or don't practice what they preach.

As a graduate student, I was enamored by artificial intelligence. I was convinced it was just a matter of time until we built a large enough computer that could emulate all of the off/on switches in our brains.

As someone living with Alzheimer's, I realize from my own first-hand experience that thinking and feeling and behaving are not functions adequately characterized or accurately emulated by an endless number of off/on switches.

I could not characterize myself as a glass or a cup or a bottle or a vessel, which acts as a barrier between me and the rest of the universe. I am an extension of my family, and they are an extension of me. I am my mother's and father's son, and they are my parents. There is more than simply leakage between a human being and his or her environment. I am never half full or half empty, I am always me. And I can never be accurately characterized as having observable, distinct, and mutually exclusive levels of anything within me (apologies to fellow psychologists and our second cousins once removed, the psychiatrists).

I am always becoming, always resisting, always embracing, and always influenced by my past. Alzheimer's disease does not change this. Forget this half full/half empty stuff—it is as useful as asking me if I am a Pentium 3 or a Pentium 4.

For those readers who know their "type" from the results of the Myers-Briggs test (I am an
ENTJ), here are some possible responses by type to the question:

*Is the glass half empty or half full?*

INTJ: Glass is made from silicon dioxide, heated to a temperature of . . .

INTP: The glass is full—half water, half air!

ENTP: Voila! 0.157 L of dihydrogen oxide, prepared by micro-gnomes.

ENTJ: Hey! This is a beer glass, not a water glass!

INFJ: This glass of water is a metaphor for my life.

INFP: But look! A crystalline vessel, filled with shimmering, life-giving nectar!

ENFP: Whooeee! Water fight!

ENFJ: There's more than enough for friends to share.

ISFJ thinks: I bet my friend would like to have some water right now . . .

ISFP (Holds up glass of water, tilts it from side to side, wiggles finger in it, licks finger, grins
    slightly, moves on.)

ESFP: There's a glass of water! You know, it's healthy to drink a lot of water! Why, I remember
    when I was growing up, we used to . . .

ESFJ: I can't believe someone would leave this dirty glass out here! Clean up this mess right
    now!

ISTJ: It's half empty now, and it wouldn't surprise me if it dried up completely.

ISTP: So? It's water. Big deal!

ESTP: You call that a glass of water? Why, back where I come from . . .

ESTJ: Hey! Whose job was it to fill up this glass?

*http://soli.inav.net/~catalyst/Humor/full.htm*

# The Flesh Is Weak(er),
# but My Spirit Is (Still) Strong

*The spirit is willing but the flesh is weak*
—Matthew 26:41

Did something/someone enter my mind the first time I took a breath of polluted Jackson Park Hospital air (that is where I was born, in Chicago, Illinois—South Side, 71st and Stony Island)? When one of my dad's sperm made a successful move on one of my mom's eggs and he scored . . . was there something more in the shell than my dad's and mom's contributions? Do I have a spirit in me that grows and shrinks (*His spirit was weakened when he saw that* . . . ), comes and goes (*He has lost his spirit because* . . . ), can be killed and resurrected (*His spirit was reborn when* . . . ), actually divides itself into pieces and enters the bodies of others (*His spirit lives on in* . . . ), is changed by Alzheimer's disease?

Having exhausted self-exploration of the impact of my disease on my religious beliefs and feelings, which are currently few, conflicted, vague, contradictory, and unorganized, I now turn to the subject of my spirit. Leaving God (in various forms and names) out of the exploration, is the sum of the parts of my plaque-filled brain greater than all its parts (plaque-filled or not)? When I roll over in our bed and look into the eyes of my spouse, laugh with my granddaughters, take my dog for a walk on a crystal clear night, listen to Mozart most any time—is there something in me that responds to my experience which is not me in a physical sense but is me in some nonphysical sense? When I heard the words, "You have early-onset dementia of the Alzheimer's type," was there something in me that started to cry before I did? And, perhaps it is still crying.

At last, to those last series of questions I have an unequivocal answer: yes and no. Yes, I believe I have a spirit. Yes, I believe it has been bruised by the knowledge that I have Alzheimer's disease. Yes, I believe I am sensing its presence more and more within me.

No, I can't describe it in rational and physical terms. I don't know where it is in my body. I don't know the physical effect Alzheimer's has upon it. I can't think about it the way I think about most "things."

With apologies to René Descartes, "I feel it all the time, therefore it is." I know it is I, because it perfectly reflects what I think, feel, and know. Yet, it has the capacity to carry me, mostly through feelings to sensations, which I cannot through the power of my own rationality control or achieve. It is an extension of me and it is me, both at the same time. I honestly believe it is an evolving part of all human beings. It just has not evolved sufficiently for us to fully appreciate and understand. However, just because it is under our rational radar screens does not mean it is not there. My own limits, plus about 10, defines the limits or possibilities of my spirit. Ten *what,* I do not know. I do know my spirit is able to pull me to depths, raise me to heights, and lead me to appreciating experiences in ways I would be unable to experience were I limited just to my intellectual abilities. It is said that most people die the way they lived. If they were generous in life, so too in death. If they were insensitive with their wives and children, so they will approach death in the same manner. I think this is also true of my spirit. It evolves as I evolve, and the pronouncement that some disease is gumming up my brain does not in and of itself dramatically influence the possibilities of change for my spirit.

# Will the Real
## Dr. Alzheimer Please Stand Up?

Once upon a time, in a country far, far away from where we are living today, there was a TV show called *What's My Line?* Three or four people would introduce themselves as the same person, and a panel of semi-celebrities would ask questions of each of them and try to establish who was the real person and which ones were the imposters. If all the celebrities misidentified the named person, the imposters could split up to and including $100!

As I jump from site to site and room to room on the Web, I have taken the nom de plume *Dr. Alzheimer.* It gets people's attention, identifies my general reason for being there, and is vaguely related to the fact that I have a Ph.D. and can legally call myself *Doctor* (even if it is only of Philosophy). Who we are is not who we say we are, especially if all others have to go on is our last name or screen name. After all, how many "hot" women and "well endowed" males can there be in the world? In addition, what are the odds of them all being in the same chat room at the same time?

Yet, when you associate your person with the word *Alzheimer,* it produces some interesting and predictable "pictures" in the minds of your readers.

You are old, at least older than they are. You have more white or gray hair than they do. You walk slightly bent over and at a slower pace than they do. You can't hear as well as they do. You surely can't understand polysyllabic words, and compound or complex sentences are confusing to you. You probably do not remember the names of your grandchildren. There is little sense in asking you your address, and listening to you babble in response to their questions is pretty much a waste of time—although they will always smile at you while you are babbling. Surely, this is a gross exaggeration of everyone's response, and it is based upon my experience. Also, based upon my experience, this is how some people, at some time, will respond to the association of the word *Alzheimer* with you or me.

When I meet new folks on the Web and they see my screen name, they are sometimes perplexed as to who I am and why the *h-e-double hockey sticks* I call myself *Dr. Alzheimer.*

Within a family, we are sometimes more who we really are than we are willing to show the rest of the world. On a good day, I am outspoken, don't always take things as seriously as others, and frequently have a slightly oblique view of common situations that others don't always find funny, interesting, true, and/or sometimes understandable. I have been diagnosed with Alzheimer's for almost three years now. I was a clinical and organizational psychologist. When I was first diagnosed, I retired from my practice and gravitated to a place where Alzheimer's-like behavior is not noticed, where those who don't have Alzheimer's act forgetful, like they don't always understand what is going on, like they have a mind independent from most other minds, like they are sometimes out of touch with what others are in touch with and in touch with what others are out of touch with, and where people sometimes don't dress or bathe like others or react to others as others do to them: I joined the academic community and started teaching. One day, I passed an evaluation form to my assistant; it was blank, and I thought I had completed it. That was the day I retired from teaching. I now work to start up chat rooms for caregivers and those for whom they care. I have a personal goal of speaking to every physician in Houston, Texas, concerning my treatment. I want to publish a book of my reactions to primarily the health care community to me and my disease. I am on the local board of directors of our Alzheimer's Association, among other activities. Most importantly, I play with my granddaughters, now 5 and 12, every day.

> *When I meet new folks on the Web and they see my screen name, they are sometimes perplexed as to who I am and why the H.E.-double hockey sticks I call myself* Dr. Alzheimer.

> *I have a personal goal of speaking to every physician in Houston, Texas.*

I think and write down what I am thinking about a lot. Some say I think and worry too much; others say my thoughts are insightful and useful to them; others say they have their own thoughts, thank you, and move on to their favorite part of life's newspaper.

Trust me, I know I am not Dr. Alzheimer. In fact, he was a physician caught in the medical paradigms of his day. The patient he treated, whose brain biopsy was used to discover the disease, was treated when she was alive as a mentally ill, difficult to manage, old, demented woman. He was almost exclusively interested in the physiology of the newly discovered disease. He spent long hours with medical students, peering into microscopes with a cigar in the corner of his mouth. The mark of how much he liked a medical student was determined by the number of cigar butts in the ashtray next to the student's microscope.

I am on a mission to provide firsthand feedback about how I feel and what I think to those who treat me and those who take care of me. It helps me to continue to feel good about myself to talk about my condition and myself. I miss parts of myself that others hear and see. I confuse recollections of conversations I did and did not have. I need more feedback from others. They need more feedback from me. My experience is increasingly different from the perceptions of others. They need to know that, and so do I. We both need to learn on the fly how to continue to figure out life, each other, and ourselves. Life is always different from day to day. Over the course of days, weeks, and years, I miss more and more of the differences. I am now more aware of them. There are differences with which I have never had to deal. Life is not only different; it is different in a different way.

Thank heavens for Dr. Alzheimer. He was the first to begin to understand me, or at least to understand me when I was dead. Now I am working on the *alive* part of understanding me in a joint venture with my caregivers.

I want to be one of a million Dr. Alzheimers.

# "Alzheimer's Disease. Alzheimer's Disease. Alzheimer's Disease!"

So, what's the big deal about saying the word *Alzheimer's*? "Alzheimer's, Alzheimer's, Alzheimer's." There—I said and wrote it three times. Why do both caregivers and their loved ones turn themselves inside out when the words *Alzheimer's disease* are mentioned? I had a friend in an early-onset group who referred to herself as "a little tipped," but she never acknowledged she had Alzheimer's disease. I know several people who faded into the fog of end-stage Alzheimer's disease never having acknowledged they had the disease in the first place. I have heard caregivers talk amongst themselves and refer to the disease as "the problem" or "you know what."

I first heard the word uttered by my general practitioner, and referring to—of all people—ME! Of course, I knew he was not talking about *me*, so it had little impact, even though I was the only other human being in the room besides him when he said it. I went to a neurologist who is a good friend of mine, and he was very careful not to use the word *Alzheimer's* to my face, because he did not feel comfortable saying it until he was sure of his diagnosis. Next, I spent two days in neuropsychological testing. I think they ran out of tests from their library and finally had to stop. Two weeks later, while working with a client in my office, I received a call from the psychologist's office telling me the report was ready. Foolishly, I said, "Fax it right over here."

To this day, three years later, I can see, hear, smell, and feel the fax paper as it came out of the machine one page at a time. In spite of my own, and the disease's, best efforts, I can still vividly remember the conclusions on the last page: *In my judgment, based upon his test results, Richard clearly has dementia, probably of the Alzheimer's type. Richard and his family should immediately contact the local Alzheimer's Association, make the necessary legal preparations, and seek to join a group through the Association.* I was numbed when I saw the words. I abruptly concluded my session, got in my car, and drove home. I called my wife, who was at work, and read her the conclusions; neither of us responded. I hung up the phone, poured myself a stiff glass of orange juice, and began to cry. Honestly, I don't know if I cried that hard on hearing the news that my mom and dad had died, but I do know I cannot cry any harder than I did that day. I rushed outside into my backyard and cried not harder, but louder. This went on for about half an hour until I literally collapsed in my garden, crushing three pepper plants in the process.

I know from graduate school that words are not the things they describe. They are symbols. They are very personal maps of territory most of us have never seen or walked through. Other words have told us what the territory is like—words from people who have experienced the territory firsthand, secondhand, thirdhand, or read it in a book, or saw it on TV, or knew of someone who knew someone who had a next-door neighbor whose mother had walked over that territory herself.

> *I called my wife, who was at work, and read her the conclusions; neither of us responded. I hung up the phone, poured myself a stiff glass of orange juice, and began to cry.*

Why, then, is this such a powerful word in our language in our society? I think that, for most people, Alzheimer's disease means certain death before your "natural time," preceded by a period of time during which you have been stripped of your personality and your memories and have become someone you cannot imagine. You have no dignity and no sense of self, and eventually you just sit around waiting for your body to forget how to keep itself alive.

Admittedly, that is a lot of territory to squeeze into the words *Alzheimer's disease*. It certainly is more than just the last name of a physician who first identified the disease through an autopsy of one of his patients. He never really wanted the disease to assume his name. Over time it just sort of happened. The same thing happened to Dr. Joseph Guillotine. He was searching for a more humane way for the death sentence to be administered. He found the slow death by hanging, or by tearing people apart limb from limb, to be inhumane. He discovered a guillotine-like machine from reading a history of executions in England. There is ample evidence to support the contention that he did not want to be remembered as the "father of the guillotine." Dr. Alois Alzheimer likely did not want to be associated forever with this disease.

I believe effort should be focused on opening up everyone involved to the issues and problems which will inevitably confront them. It should not be a question of whether people will say or use the word, but whether they will talk about the territory they believe (inaccurately or accurately) the word describes. I have been in groups in which the caregiver or the leader gives it his or her best shot to get the loved one to say, "I have Alzheimer's disease." Now, what that means to them, versus what it means to the person saying it, is lost in a tug-of-war over saying the word.

To most, *dementia* is a scary word all by itself. We do not want to grow old, and we're not growing old like other people our age seem to be. And, after all, "60 really isn't *that* old," say people who just turned 60. I believe that the words *dementia* and *Alzheimer's* are, for most people, variations of the same thing in their minds. "Alzheimer's is just a really bad case of dementia." Those of us in the know know we're talking about two different territories; but, even for us, it's scary to imagine ourselves living in either territory.

I believe we should be less concerned with the words we use to describe our health (our territory) and focus more on an effort to understand what we mean when we use certain words. How close are caregivers and their loved ones to understanding what the same word means? What do we need to do in order for us all to agree that this is what the word means? Its impact on each of us may be different, and that is one thing we can agree on.

> *We think we can control our fear of the territory by controlling the saying of the word. If I do not say I am pregnant, does that mean I am not pregnant?*

Some words are so powerful because the territory we believe it describes is so scary, is so scandalous, is so sinful, is so gross that we believe if we do not use the word, then we won't think about the territory. In these cases, we have already linked the symbol (the word) and the territory (its meaning). We think we can control our fear of the territory by controlling the saying of the word. If I do not say I am pregnant, does that mean I am not pregnant?

Please, sit down with each other and talk first about the territory. Nothing is to be gained, and much will be lost, if saying the words aloud so traumatizes those involved that they do not hear what follows the words *Alzheimer's disease.*

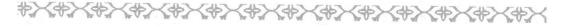

When *people with Alzheimer's disease* are concerned about stigma, a diagnosis of Alzheimer's disease occurrs on average 3.5 years (40.1 months) after symptoms appear.

When *caregivers* are concerned about stigma, delay of diagnosis is even more severe, averaging 6 years (71.4 months).

*http://www.kusi.com/health/2499656.html*

# Am I My Brain? Or Is My Brain Me?

If René Descartes was right, and our existence is determined, confirmed, and maintained by the fact that we are thinking—"I think, therefore I am"—then is how I think and what I think *who* I am, beyond simply existing? Lots of people claim that their heart and what is in it defines who they are. Others define themselves as young or old by the functionality of various organs. I have the kidneys of a 30-year-old, the sexual stamina and appetite of a 22-year-old man (or a 32-year-old woman), the eyes of an octogenarian, the lungs of an athlete. Is who I am really defined by the shape, length, weight, condition, and contents of one or more of my organs? Or is what differentiates me, what defines me as a human being, something more than the physical parameters of my organs, bones, and skin?

For those of us with brains infected with some form of dementia, are we really the same people we were prior to the onset of dementia? Is there something or someone that is mutually exclusive and to which we refer as "the disease?" As the disease consumes more and more of our brains, is it also consuming more and more of us? Who we are? *If* we really are?

After they have spent years dealing with the impact of end-stage Alzheimer's on their loved ones, I have heard caregivers say out loud, "It would be best for him if he died in his sleep. Mercifully, it should happen sooner rather than later."

Wait a minute here! Can we talk about this before you increase my pain medication? Pull the plug? Withdraw drugs, food, or water? What happened to me and the disease being separate entities? Am I now less human? Is my existence diminishing in lockstep and because of the progression of the disease? Is my existence less and less important because my shrinking brain is more and more filled with the tangled plaques and dead cells caused by Alzheimer's disease?

Is there still a "Richard" who is mutually exclusive from the disease? Who am I after

> *Wait a minute here! Can we talk about this before you increase my pain medication? Pull the plug?*

others, who I know still love me, are starting to think positively about it maybe being best for me if I ceased to exist?

Is there nothing left of Richard, just a shell filled with Alzheimer's disease? Does Stage 3 or 7 or however the end-stage is clinically described, signify the loss of self and victory for the disease?

Okay, so maybe I should stop asking questions and propose some answers, at least for myself. On good days, and for me those are still most days, I agree with the caregiver who says, "It's a philosophical argument of the type that creates jobs for individuals who still insist on majoring in philosophy. This is not the Richard I knew. He would not know or appreciate himself if he could return to a pre-Alzheimer's time and observe himself as he is today. This is not who Richard wanted to be, how he wanted the 'twilight moments' of his life to transpire. The way he sits there, the way he looks, the fact that he is unable to take care of himself in any way, shape, or form—this is simply not Richard! He has lost his sense of dignity, his sense of himself, his apparent awareness of others, especially his loved ones."

> *I have no idea who I will be when I am wheeled out for the final act on the Alzheimer's stage. But, I do know I will* be . . . *I will still be me . . . perhaps a* me *different from what I have ever been before.*

I have no idea who I will be when I am wheeled out for the final act on the Alzheimer's stage. But, I do know I will *be* . . . I will still be me . . . perhaps a *me* different from what I have ever been before. The issue is this: When I become someone other than the *me* we all know and many love; when I am physically unable to end my own life, should I even want to; when the ultimate responsibility for keeping me alive is neither mine nor my health care provider's, should we agree now on how my caregivers should act on my behalf?

As my "thirty-something" friends would say, "Let's have a conversation." In fact, it is worth conversing about this at regular intervals until I can no longer follow the conversation.

# Good Habits and Mindless Patterns

The other day, I looked up from my desk and it was 5:00 P.M. Now, that in and of itself is not worth commenting on. Unfortunately, the previous time I could recall was 10 A.M. What happened in the missing seven hours of my life? Alzheimer's disease sometimes saps my initiative to maintain awareness of each moment, each minute, each hour. In place of conscious behaviors, I have developed patterns—groups of repetitive behaviors that are mostly formed and reinforced by external influences. They do not necessarily accomplish anything; they are simply repeated over and over again. After a while, you can remove the external influences (the clock on my desk) and I still stop working at noon and eat lunch, even if I am not particularly hungry. I still take the dog for a walk at 10, 4, and 9, even if she does not need or want to walk.

Habits, on the other hand, are ways of accomplishing objectives that work efficiently, effectively, and are relatively easy to do. Habits, in my way of thinking (such as it is), are the means you apply to some task to achieve some end or goal. I still know what good habits are. I still practice them once in a while. But the patterns of my life, the things I seem to do and not do as a result of the disease, seem to be edging out the good habits that used to define how I acted in most of my waking hours. I was good at managing my time. I was good at writing down goals and objectives and the timelines to meet them. I was good at leading a purposeful life. I no longer apply good habits to my activities, because I no longer have purposeful activities. I have fallen into meaningless patterns; not all of the time, of course, but more than in the past.

Time does not mean much to me now. I do not know and I seldom care if it is Monday or Wednesday or Sunday. I do not know if it is 10 A.M., 1 P.M., or 4 P.M. I do not know if it is January 1 or February 15 or March 13. I do not care. It does not make a difference in my life.

I continue to make lists of things to do, most of which I do not do. None of these lists achieves a goal! None of these lists supports an objective that, in turn, achieves a goal. I have day lists, week lists, partial day lists (sometimes two or three), and the ultimate—I now have lists of lists. They are color coded and different sizes; some

> *I have day lists, week lists, partial day lists (sometimes two or three), and the ultimate—I now have lists of lists.*

stick up by themselves, and others have holes punched in them for hanging.

There are things I have to do to get through the day. The list tells me to do this and that, arrange for this and that, call or write this or that person. They detail a never-ending list of doctor's appointments, occasional needs from the food store, and chores around the house, most of which I either forget to do or do poorly. I'm not as clear as I formerly was concerning the purpose of my life, and I don't live as much of my life feeling as if I was driven and moving with and toward a vision of who I wanted to be. My life now is not a mission, with goals and objectives of how I want to get there. I am wandering around, lost in an unfamiliar forest, with no expectation of ever being able to find my home again. Moreover, I do not seem to care!

My good habits moved me forward, but mindless activities keep me stuck. Given what is going on between my ears, perhaps being stuck is the best I can hope for.

# "You Sure Don't Talk Like You Have Alzheimer's." (The Great Pretender)

What do The Platters,* Pedro the Great,** and Richard all have in common? They have all been viewed by some as "a great pretender." To this day, well-intended friends and family still say to me, "You sure don't seem like you have Alzheimer's disease to me." They say and mean this, I believe, as a positive observation and comment. "You act normal, just like me!"

I don't know what to say or how to act when I am confronted with this statement. The longer I live with this disease, the briefer the periods of time I feel "normal." Previously, I could easily lapse back into my prediagnosis ways of feeling and thinking. Now, my thinking almost continually reminds me that I am not normal. Because thinking determines feelings, I almost always feel like I am not normal. Of course I realize that *normal* is a relative term, but I try harder and harder every day to outwardly appear normal. The unintended consequence of this strategy is that I am constantly reminded that I am not normal and must try harder and harder to appear so.

> *Of course I realize that* normal *is a relative term, but I try harder and harder every day to outwardly appear normal.*

Richard appears to have been able to more or less effectively compensate for his cognitive decline with his superior verbal abilities and crystallized knowledge. His relative strength in his verbal abilities may make it difficult to observe impairment on a typical neurological mental status evaluation. His verbal abilities, along with compensatory strategies, and effective medication management have allowed him to function within normal limits until recently. Despite this report,

*Recorded the song "The Great Pretender"; lyrics and music by Buck Ram.
**The major character in the play *Pedro de Urdemalas* (Pedro, the Great Pretender) by Miguel de Cervantes, who is best known as the author of *Don Quixote de la Mancha*.

> Richard appears to use his verbal abilities and charismatic personality to advocate for continued independence (e.g., driving alone). However, findings of this evaluation suggest impairment in many cognitive domains that likely result in a significantly reduced ability in activities of daily living, leading to reduced functioning on a daily basis.
>
> —Psychological Assessment Report 6/1/04

I never was sure about his claim that I possessed a "charismatic personality," but I am increasingly aware of my conscious use of language to compensate for my diminishing cognitive abilities. When I was in the eighth grade, I read *30 Days to a More Powerful Vocabulary*. When I was a debater in college, it was part of the "debate speak" culture to use polysyllabic words. When I studied communication and psychology, I understood how and why there is so much power in the words we use to describe and, in fact, prescribe our reality. General Semantics and Albert Ellis showed me how words are used as maps, how maps are used as territories, how territories are treated as all-inclusive, and how they all generate and influence our feelings.

You won't see a picture of me in this book putting on my shirt inside out. It happens many times a week. You won't hear me fishing for a word, because I have time to pause when writing. It happens, many times per day. You won't see me wandering around, not knowing or caring where I am. I look and sound "normal."

So how come I can write a book if I have Alzheimer's disease? How can I seem to some, sometimes, as a normal person? I so much want it not to be true that I have this disease that I pretend to all, including myself, that I don't. On a mostly subconscious level, I have learned to distract others and myself from my shortcomings, and shift and maintain focus on my strengths. Don't we all do this?

---

The song, *The Great Pretender*, became identified with the music group The Platters. Martha, the widow of one of the original Platters, sued the only remaining member of the group, Herb, who still sings with a group called The Platters. She wanted exclusive rights to call the group she was managing *The Platters*. She lost. According to the law, she was the pretender and not Herb. Pretending never seems to stop!

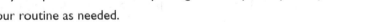

# DEALING WITH THE DIAGNOSIS

Finding out that a loved one has Alzheimer's disease can be stressful, frightening, and overwhelming. As you begin to take stock of the situation, here are some tips that may help:

- Ask the doctor any questions you have about AD. Find out what treatments might work best to alleviate symptoms or address behavior problems.

- Contact organizations such as the Alzheimer's Association and the Alzheimer's Disease Education and Referral (ADEAR) Center for more information about the disease, treatment options, and caregiving resources. Some community groups may offer classes to teach caregiving, problem-solving, and management skills.

- Find a support group where you can share your feelings and concerns. Members of support groups often have helpful ideas or know of useful resources based on their own experiences. Online support groups make it possible for caregivers to receive support without having to leave home.

- Study your day to see if you can develop a routine that makes things go more smoothly. Keep in mind that the way the person functions may change from day to day, so try to be flexible and adapt your routine as needed.

- Consider using adult day care or respite services to ease the day-to-day demands of caregiving.

- Begin to plan for the future. This may include getting financial and legal documents in order, investigating long-term care options, and determining what services are covered by health insurance and Medicare.

# "Knock Knock"

(Knock knock)

Gregory: Mr. Taylor, remember me, I'm Gregory, the fourth grader you bought some wrapping paper from last month. I'm here to deliver it now.

Richard: Great!

(Parents get out of car, each with two shopping bags full of over-priced gift wrapping paper, rolls of tape which I could purchase for a fraction of the price at the local dollar store, and two pairs of special cutting shears [which brings the number of special cutting shears in our house to four].)

Gregory: My mom says you owe me $102.55.

Richard: No problem. Linda, I need a check. Where is the checkbook?

Linda: (speaking from the backyard) Why do you need the checkbook?

Richard: I just need one check. Where is the checkbook?

Linda: It's in the kitchen, but I will have to come in and get it myself.

Richard: Just tell me where the checkbook is; I only need one check.

Linda: It's somewhere in the kitchen. I told you already, I have to come in and get it myself.

Richard: I'm standing in the kitchen; just tell me where to look.

Linda: It's too complicated. Just give me a minute to finish out here and I'll be in to help you.

Richard: I have a little boy at the front door waiting for a check.

Linda: Did you buy more of something we already have from some kid we don't know?

Richard: Maybe. I just need the checkbook.

Linda: I'm coming in right now.

Parents: Hello, we are Gregory's parents. We just wanted to thank you. Gregory won the prize for selling the largest single order.

Richard: Oh?

Linda: Every kid does who comes here selling something and runs into my husband.

124

Richard:   May I please have the checkbook?
Linda:    I'll write the check, but I want you to know I am not happy
          about this happening again and again.

Understand, I haven't written a check in over two years. It was a big deal
for me to be able to write a check. Of course, it would have also delayed
discussing the issue of why I purchased $102.55 worth of gift wrapping.

My spouse would tell you I have become careless and extrava-
gant with money. I always want more. I have no sense of how we are
going to pay for our future once she retires.

Is it me or is it the disease that caused me to decide to order so
much wrapping paper? Was this an example of me still trying to prove
to myself that I'm okay and can make my own decisions? Was I just
charmed by Gregory? Or did I just not realize the total price of the
materials I ordered? (I might add, my wife
carries a red pencil in her car and, amazingly
enough, most of what she buys is marked down
with red pencil.)

As with most behaviors in life, a single
clear intent is not as easy to establish as
one would wish (B.F. Skinner notwithstand-
ing). Life is gray, and intent is grayer. I am
turning darker gray every day! It must be
very difficult now for my caregivers, who once thought they knew me,
to figure me out and act accordingly. Sometimes, I'm glad I'm not
them. Increasingly, I wish I weren't me!

> *Is it me or is it the disease that caused me to decide to order so much wrapping paper?*

---

The hippocampus takes our immediate thoughts and impressions and turns them into memories. Alzheimer's attacks the hippocampus first, so short-term memory is the first thing to
fail. Eventually, new memories become impossible to make and learning is a thing of the past.
Without knowing what just happened, it's difficult for people to judge things like time, place,
and what's going on around them.

*http://www.pbs.org/theforgetting/symptoms/index.html#brain*

# What Will I Do Today?

How does it happen so quickly? What is the process? Can it be stopped? Reversed? At least not encouraged? How does a competent, independent, fully functioning adult morph into someone who sits passively in a chair by the side of the road, apparently watching the world pass by between meals and naps? How does an adult who is working eight or more hours a day transform into someone sitting at home waiting for "I can't remember her name? The nice lady who gives away cars, or was it books or snacks? I can't remember exactly. Oh well, it doesn't really matter, I'll watch whatever is on the TV."

I'll tell you how it is happening to me and a few of my friends. We were talking about this very subject the other day. I mentioned how frustrating it is for me since I stopped driving. Now I am always dependent on someone else to decide when and where I am going, if it requires a car to get there. At first, I just asked people for a ride and told them where I wanted to go. They almost always said "Yes, but. . . . " They didn't have the time right now, but they would certainly do it soon or on the weekend. When the weekend came, I asked them again and then we argued about if what I wanted to get was necessary, or could they get it for me, or what was the big rush. And, why did I wait to the last minute to ask for things? Didn't I realize they had families, jobs, and lives to live, too?

That's when I decided to start to keep a list on the kitchen table of things I need and things I want to do that require the support of others. My caregivers would consult this list from time to time. Sometimes, they ran an errand for me, and suddenly a bottle of Heinz ketchup showed up in the refrigerator without me having to go to the store and get it. Great!? But then I discovered that I never went grocery shopping. In fact I would go weeks without getting away from my house! I had to write everything I needed on the list and others would buy it for me, maybe. If they thought I didn't need it, or it was too expensive, I didn't get it. One day, I did accompany someone to the store, and it felt wonderful to be able to walk up and down the aisles and buy things based on impulse. Wow, shopping is fun—I forgot how much.

Waiting time and the percentage of items never received diminished and all seemed well; that is, for groceries. If I needed something for a project on which I was working, I wrote it on the list and politely waited. Sooner or later, it usually showed up on the kitchen table. Not always the brand I would have purchased, not always exactly as I wanted it, but it was close enough. My projects had to wait for others to purchase the necessary materials. One day, I accompanied someone to Builder's Square (or was it Lowe's or Home Depot?), and it felt wonderful to walk up and down the aisles and compare products on my own, to get new ideas of things to do. I was free to be an adult again, if only for a short time.

> *One day, I did accompany someone to the store, and it felt wonderful to be able to walk up and down the aisles and buy things based on impulse.*

Every morning when I wake up, I try to organize my day. I scratch a few notes on one of 57 pads of paper I keep around the house to make lists of things so I don't forget to do them. Unfortunately, for me, much of what I plan to do is dependent upon others' cooperation that day.

I look at my list and say to myself: "This is too confusing. I don't understand that. I've gotten frustrated in the past when I did this. I need to go somewhere to get materials. I need someone to watch me do this to make sure I don't hurt myself . . ." Unfortunately, the possibilities for needing help are limitless. So what am I going to do today? Am I to do what others think I should do that day? Should I sit around and wait for others to tell me what I am to do that day? Perhaps I should awaken not wanting to do anything, and then be surprised when I accomplish something at the prodding of others and with the help of others. One way of looking at it is that it really doesn't make any difference what I do today, because I can do it tomorrow.

People are no longer dependent on me to do something for them, I am dependent on them. People don't wait for me to accomplish something for them, I wait for them to accomplish something for me. I'm not helpless. I can do things on my own. Increasingly, however, doing things on my own runs the risk of doing them wrong either for me or for others—or maybe not doing things at all. What will I do today? More and more, I wait.

# Drifting Away from
# My Head and into My Heart

⚿⚿⚿⚿⚿⚿

Some mornings, after I've had a handful of pills, a glass of orange juice, and a piece of fruit, I come into my office, sit at my desk, turn on my computer, and discover I have nothing of import to say or write. So I read my e-mail. I check for spyware. I make a few phone calls. I send a few e-mails. And I still have nothing of import to say or write. What I do have are barrels and barrels full of feelings—some of them toxic, some of them happy, some of them sad—and barrels and barrels full of mixed feelings. The locus of my attention is definitely shifting from my head to my heart. I feel and think about feelings more than I think about thinking. I feel sad, and mad, and happy, and grateful. I feel loved, ignored, needed, and like a dying albatross that is chained around each of the people who cares about me. Sometimes I'm very happy, and sometimes I'm very sad, and at all times I am aware of all my feelings. It's as if the feelings I was long able to keep on separate hangers in my closet (the one with the door to which only I had the key) now have all been woven into one heavy cloak that covers me from head to foot.

One reason I live in my feelings is because I have grown weary of thinking about myself and my future. I'm tired of trying to figure it out, because I am in a constant state of flux. There is no consistent figuring, because I keep switching the base I am using to determine the value of the numbers I'm trying to figure out. One moment I am in base 10, familiar to me since grammar school, and the next moment I am in a base I do not recognize and whose rules I do not and probably cannot understand. So what do I use to fuel the blast furnace of intellectual curiosity, self-exploration, and the need to know which has defined me for the past 60 or so years?

Send in the clowns. Send in my feelings. Send in my past, my present, and my future stripped of rational considerations and baring all of my naked feelings.

For years, I believed my feelings were actually slaves of my thoughts. Every true-believing rational-emotive therapist will tell you that feelings are responses to thoughts. So when you feel as if your feelings are out of control, what does that say about your thought process? And when your thought process becomes irrational, unpredictable, and out of control, what happens to your feelings?

> *I, like most human beings, am very good at hiding my thoughts but not so good at hiding my feelings.*

Sometimes, I don't even realize the impact the disease is having on my thoughts until I sit down and think about what happened. Almost always, others know its impact through my inappropriate or surprising expression of feelings. I, like most human beings, am very good at hiding my thoughts but not so good at hiding my feelings. So in spite of what your neuropsychological testing may tell you, the first outward sign of the disease is probably revealed through your feelings.

These writings are not in exact chronological order, so please read them as independent, standalone moments in my life. If I sometimes contradict what I said on a previous page, it may not necessarily be the next day that I did so. Then again, it may be. Consistency was once one of my strong points, but alas is no longer. (R.T.)

# *Falling*

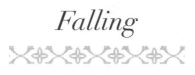

Ihave fallen off the plateau on which I was firmly standing for the past 10 or so months and I am in sort of an unconscious free fall. I just had a battery of tests comparing me to my past four years arm wrestling with Dr. Alzheimer, and he is clearly in the lead. My IQ has fallen from 148 to 114. I am in the bottom standard deviation (bottom 2% of the population who is able to even complete the tests) in short-term memory. My processing speed is slightly faster than a concrete brick, and my self-awareness is close to that of a lizard—natural reflexes working well, meta perceptive comes and goes, as does self-understanding. I can sit here and know what I want to do and do something completely different and not know I am doing it. It just happened. It has happened most of today.

There is more than one tear in my eye as I write this because I know I am entering the darkness of Alzheimer's disease. I can still see what others see, sometimes. I miss it, sometimes. Sometimes I see something no one else sees, but still sometimes I can see what others see. I sometimes wonder if blindness isn't a better alternative to this! Not suicide, mind you; just let's gets on with it.

Not only don't I see, hear, touch, and feel well; what I do see takes me agonizingly long to process and understand. When I just open my mouth and respond, as I did in the past, my chances of saying something wrong, inappropriate, hurtful, and/or confusing to my listeners increases every day!

It is increasingly more difficult for my caregivers to understand me or what is going on within and with me. I know this from their tears, anger, and frustration. I cannot understand or appreciate it myself when "it" (whatever it represents) is happening! Afterwards my reevaluation of whatever it is does not make much difference. The harm has been done, the mistakes have been made, and the feelings have been tromped on.

I am weary of trying to understand others and myself. The information I now use to understand my world and me is faulty, as are my conclusions. What is the use of even trying to understand or make rational decisions when you do not have accurate perceptions, recollections, or information? Feelings of insecurity undermine even the most confident of my conclusions. I can better appreciate why some allow and encourage themselves to quickly slip away from the here and now, and embrace their own versions of here and now. It's tempting. It's surely easier. Living in and for the moment assumes the ability to know what is going on, what I am doing in any given moment. I don't always know either! Going with the flow assumes there is a flow, not a series of abrupt starts and stops.

Losing the ability to accurately think about myself, to confidently know what I am doing, to have some clues as to how and why I feel as I do—as I understand and accept this is who I now am and it's not going to get any better—what is left for me to enjoy in myself and my surroundings?

# Will the Real Richard Taylor
# Ever Reveal Himself to Me?

I am not who you thought I was. I am not who you wish I was. I am someone who, even I am increasingly discovering, I don't know. I don't claim that I was entirely familiar with who I was, but I know for sure I am less familiar with who I am than who I was.

I have changed. I am changing. I don't like it any more than you do. In fact, I probably dislike the change even more than you, because I seem to have almost no control over who I am becoming. Frankly, sometimes I feel like I have little or no control over who I am. I argue more and listen less. I jump to conclusions, and I am sometimes fearful to express my opinion. Doesn't sound like the Richard you and I knew, does it?

This personal change phenomenon is, in my humble opinion, the most powerful and devastating symptom of dementia I have thus far experienced. There is little written about it, other than to say, "There may be personality changes." I may become a tad "more confrontational, paranoid, confused" than I was before Dr. Alzheimer took up residence in my brain. Where are the studies of these phenomena? Where are the books, the papers, the programs on what to expect, how to deal with it, what pills to take to reverse it? Who is researching the "Alzheimer's personalities syndromes?"

And while I am complaining, what about the changes in my caregivers' personalities? Simply saying, "Your loved one has Alzheimer's disease" triggers fear and deeply buried attitudes and beliefs that guarantee personality changes in even the most stable of individuals.

Researchers are almost down to studying the movement of individual quarks and charms as they unpredictably bounce around in the brains of individuals diagnosed with dementia of the Alzheimer's type, yet no one seems to know or care about the what, when, where, and why of what happens to the personalities of individuals diagnosed with the disease. Broad generalizations of what may and may not happen to our personalities certainly predict and capture some of the changes but are of little practical use to those of us living with the changes.

When I was in graduate school, I became fascinated by artificial intelligence. I was confident that if we just had a big enough computer, we would be able to replicate human thought. Freud seemed to believe if we could just get the three cranky elves living between our ears, who were self-centered and constantly defensive about their own point of view, to get along with each other, we could all live more predictable and happy lives. Skinner was confident that if only we had a long enough list of behaviors and what preceded them and what followed them, we could predict human behavior. Others thought that we need only look at the driver's license of a person; once their date of birth was verified, we could understand them because we'd know their life stage.

Thus far, "normal" brains have resisted all attempts to describe them in a manner that could impose predictability on their internal actions and the behaviors they produce. Let Dr. Alzheimer, or Dr. Lewy, or any of the other diseases of dementia tromp around someone's brain, and the result is more than unpredictable. It produces something that cannot be described and predicted by those who do not have a brain footprinted by dementia. How can anyone ever hope to describe the fifth or tenth dimensions (if indeed there are such things or places)? We all live and use the same tool: our brains. Even though we are still unable to understand the ecology of the brain, it is the best and only tool we have to understand and describe the ecology of a brain affected by dementia. We have yet to agree on the relationship between thought and behavior. We have only guesses as to the physical basis of an individual's personality. Little wonder that nontenured researchers aren't lining up for grants to study and understand the nature of personality change in individuals with Alzheimer's disease.

> *This personal change phenomenon is, in my humble opinion, the most powerful and devastating symptom of dementia I have thus far experienced.*

Along comes Richard Taylor, complaining that no one is trying to understand the personality changes associated with Alzheimer's disease. I acknowledge that we all are living in a dark room when it comes to describing the walls of our personality. I'm not looking for certainty at the .05 level. I'm looking for support from professionals, based on experience dealing with clients who are at least in the same boat as I, if not sitting in the same deck chair.

I want psychiatrists to put down their prescription pads for a moment and listen to me. I want psychologists to open their own minds beyond what they learned in graduate school and attempt to see me not through the eyes of someone who died years ago, but as someone who is marching not only to a different drummer but down a different road than most all of their other clients. Help me understand myself the best way I can on my own terms. Attempt to learn what my terms are *today*. Develop treatment models based on the stages of my disease, not on the stages of life as they were dreamed up in the early 20th century.

> *I want psychiatrists to put down their prescription pads for a moment and listen to me.*

If I must lose control of my cognitive process, knowing what is happening is the next best thing. If I am going to become argumentative, meaner, paranoid, and/or withdrawn, please tell me in advance why and how this will happen, and it would be nice to know when and where. I've reached the point where "unusual behavior" on my part goes unnoticed until someone points it out well after the fact. I am exasperated, embarrassed, confused, and feel increasingly helpless. I am a believer in "knowledge is power"—not necessarily the power to change myself, but the power that comes from knowing and understanding who I am in this fleeting moment, and, most important, the power to better understand and appreciate the reactions of my caregivers.

I want my caregivers to better appreciate the differences concerning how I think and what I think about. For instance, if I call you "Mom" or "Dad," I am probably not confusing you with my mom or dad; I know they are dead. I may be thinking about the feelings and behaviors I associate with mom and dad. I miss those feelings; I need them. It's just that I so closely associate those feelings with my mom and dad that the words I use become interchangeable when I talk about them. I don't take the time or I can't or won't make the distinction between the people and the feelings.

Frequently, my caregivers acknowledge that they don't understand me. Sometimes, they admit to being temporarily depressed. Always, they see me as the cause of their own problems. Oh, sure, in the beginning they said it was the disease talking. Now they don't hear the disease; they hear mostly me. Therefore, I am the cause of whatever changes they are experiencing in their own personalities. If only

I were different, they could and would be their former selves again. We could all return to the good old days: when we were all more predictable; when the unwritten rules of how to get along, how to love each other, what to say, and what not to say were all etched in our unconscious and dutifully followed by all; when we felt we knew each other and ourselves.

Surely, these disease-driven changes and the fears they produce, and the influence of the changes and fears on the stability and structure of human personality, is the most common problem my disease imposes on interpersonal dynamics and sense of self. Surely, each of the other diseases of dementia stirs up the dynamics between family, caregivers, and friends and the individual diagnosed with dementia.

I am always amazed, envious, and a tad suspicious of individuals who are also dealing with Dr. Alzheimer and proudly and loudly proclaim that the disease and its impact on them has turned their lives around in a most positive sense. "I smell more flowers. I appreciate more weather-related events (usually sunsets). I better appreciate and understand my loved ones. I have turned this lemon of a disease into naturally sweetened lemonade."

I am amazed because such has not been the case for me. Although I have a few more "peak experiences," which I naturally attribute to the increased sensitivity to life created by the diagnosis, I cannot say that this disease has brightened my relationships. They were already very bright prior to the diagnosis, and I have to say that most of them have dimmed somewhat.

I am envious because I wish I could always see a silver lining through the dark clouds shining. When I was first diagnosed, I rushed to my local Alzheimer's Association and checked out a dozen of their informational videotapes. All of them were at least 10 years old, recorded in black and white, focused on individuals in the late stages of the disease, and directed almost exclusively to caregivers. I guess the folks who find greater good in this experience didn't see those tapes.

I am a tad suspicious of their positive proclamations because it is very hard for me to even imagine human beings not sometimes feeling and actually being overwhelmed by this disease. I believe that all diseases that disrupt our thinking, our memories, or our personalities create inescapable and profound effects on us and on those who care for us. There are no self-help books, no classes, no TV shows that teach me how to deal with these profound changes in myself or in those who love and care for me. The definitive book, *What It's Really Like to Have Alzheimer's Disease,* will never be written, because soon after potential authors acquired comprehensive first-hand experience on which to base the book, they would die.

We can't make meaningful and useful rational guesses about an irrational process. My brain is not the opposite of yours—rational versus irrational. We are, each of us, captives of our own paradigms, our own minds, our own memories, our own hardware. From your perspective, I have faulty hardware. From my perspective, you have faulty hardware.

When I told my wife we could never fully appreciate each other's thoughts and feelings, she became distraught. She took it to mean I was claiming I would never be able to feel her sorrow and hurt, nor she mine. This was only partially correct. Caregivers and individuals living with the diagnosis both travel down the same Alzheimer's Boulevard; however, my lane has some different potholes in it than my wife's, and vice versa. We each are forced to take different detours. Sometimes we can walk hand in hand, and other times we are miles apart. We will each end up at different destinations. We label the trip with the same name, but in fact we are on two different journeys: Mine pulls me away from her and keeps her from walking next to me. I believe it is healthier and makes it easier for us to acknowledge this fact. We don't and can't really walk in each other's shoes. Each pair may say "Alzheimer's disease" on them, but they fit differently, they take us in different directions, and one pair wears out much quicker than the other.

> *When I told my wife we could never fully appreciate each other's thoughts and feelings, she became distraught.*

My caregivers seem to spend a great deal of time talking to each other about how I have changed. They spend even more time sharing practical suggestions on how to prevent me from hurting myself and others. (I wish they would spend twice as much time on practical suggestions to enable me to continue doing what I want to do without hurting myself or others.) They worry that I am not the person they knew me to be—the person they now wish I was. Oh, how they want me to be the husband, the dad, the friend I was (or at least the one they wanted me to be but I never quite was).

I'm not. I can't. I don't want to be, because I realize I can't go back. In my mind I just want to be myself. *Really, I want to feel like I am back in control of myself (whoever that may be at any given moment).* I don't want to get mad and then not realize it until someone comments on it a day later. I want to keep an open mind instead of letting myself be influenced by heaven-only-knows what cognitive processes. I certainly don't know why I thought this or that, or reached this or that conclusion. I want to be able to complete tasks one at a time, not seemingly wander from one half-completed task to another. I want to be able to understand things, quickly and easily. I could (*could* meaning *used to*) change the oil in my lawn mower, or rewind my weed eater, or put up my outside Christmas decorations in a flash. Now, I find myself confused as to exactly what I am doing and how I should do it. I misplace things right under my nose. I can't recall the name of the misplaced object to tell others who want to help me locate it. Names have moved from near certainty, to guessing, to not a clue.

I was, and in fact still think I am, a pretty "smart guy." *Smart* is probably the wrong word to use. I have a large vocabulary, a loud voice, and a Ph.D.—a great combination if one is trying to hide one's early-stage Alzheimer's disease. I am also tall, I have a professorial-looking grey beard, I have that impressive though increasingly inaccurate vocabulary, and—did I mention—I am quite tall. Both consciously and unconsciously, I developed some pretty slick strategies to hide my scrambled and fading cognitive functions. I would control conversations, change subjects, use words few understand (and, thus, were hesitant to question), and on and on. (Someone should research and identify the strategies folks like me use to cover up their deficiencies.) I have arrived to the point at which uncomfortable silence has replaced snappy conversation. Where a puzzled look, sometimes followed by a tear in my right eye, follows my obviously inappropriate response in conversation. I know something is wrong. Given enough time, I can analyze it and understand some, but not all, of what happened. Increasingly, however, I must live with the fact that knowing why and how has little to no impact on helping me prevent it from happening again.

> *I have a large vocabulary, a loud voice, and a Ph.D.—a great combination if one is trying to hide one's early-stage Alzheimer's disease.*

It must be harder and harder for others to go with the flow of my disease-driven personality changes, to understand me, to accept me, to love me. It certainly is for me!

We're entering an age of acceleration. The models underlying society at every level, which are largely based on a linear model of change, are going to have to be redefined. Because of the explosive power of exponential growth, the 21st century will be equivalent to 20,000 years of progress at today's rate of progress; organizations have to be able to redefine themselves at a faster and faster pace. And what about the human beings? How fast will they change? And what about people living with one of the diseases of dementia? How will this change in the external change rate impact their internal change rate? Good questions, don't you think?

# From the Outside In

# *Whose Fault Is It*
## *That I Don't Understand You?*

⋉⊕⋊⊕⋉⊕⋊⊕⋉⊕⋊

When writing, it is never my intent to convince caregivers that they should feel bad about themselves. They should not feel guilty or ashamed about their relationship with their loved one living with the disease. I do want them to know how I think and feel, from my perspective, which they can never be in a position to fully realize; I also can't ever see our interactions from their perspective.

I acknowledge that I am not always "fair" or understanding of the caregiver's situation and responsibilities. I do not always, in fact, consider "the other side of the coin." I am not writing about Alzheimer's disease and its impact on Mr. T and his caregivers. I am writing about Mr. T.'s experience with Alzheimer's disease and with his family. I don't always have a solution for myself or my reader. I don't pretend to always be reasonable. I am selfish, self-centered, and really care about my own interests. Just like each of you! Please don't take my words as personal judgments of your own behaviors. And when they are (for I too am far from perfect), see this as evidence of my humanness, not as indictments of you! If we could both exchange writings like these, and then sit down and talk to each other and truly listen to each other, we could come a long way toward at least understanding and appreciating each other, but not necessarily agreeing with each other. But, if we are ever to agree, we first need to understand and appreciate each other for who and what we perceive ourselves to be today.

When we both started this journey down Alzheimer's Boulevard, we both believed and agreed that we were on this journey together, hand in hand, as husband or wife, or daughter and father, etc. I have learned that although we believe we are on the same road, we are, in fact, confined to our own lanes. We can't cross over the double yellow line. It's not against the law; it's physically and mentally impossible. We can see each other, speak with each other, and even hold each other. Yet, we each have our own pot holes, our own detours, and our own road and life hazards that we must traverse by ourselves and within ourselves.

These differences are not trivial. The farther along the road we go, the clearer it should be that we will not arrive at the same destination, at the same time. If we don't keep this in mind, we are apt to make assumptions about what the other is thinking, needing, and wanting to make their respective journeys more comfortable, easier, and more enjoyable. We are each likely to recall what worked in the past and assume it will work now and tomorrow. We will unconsciously look for clues in each other, based on assumptions of wants and needs that simply don't apply right now and won't in the future.

These honest, well-intended behaviors may meet our need to feel like we are trying hard, doing the right things, doing everything humanly possible to support each other. In fact, though, they serve to reinforce feelings of loneliness—no one understands me, no one cares enough to listen to me or take what I say at face value. It is just as simple to understand these misperceptions as it is to understand the misperceptions of others. Some are reading a chapter from the 1999 edition of "How to Meet Richard's Wants and Needs" and Richard is reading from a new, revised paperback edition published today. This new edition is revised on a daily basis and is titled, "What Needs and Wants Do I Have and How Should Others Meet Them." Is it little wonder the twain shall never meet? They are not now parts of the same twain.

This is not a sinful situation. It's not worthy of self-loathing, public confessions of stupidity, private confessions of personal failure, worthlessness, or feelings of depression and anxiety. As long as there is no intent to ignore what we know to be the truth or to mistreat each other, we should forgive ourselves for not being perfect and move forward. We must seek more information from each other, so we can more effectively share feelings and try to meet each others' needs and wants.

We should listen to each other *as we speak today*. Take what we say, as best we can, at face value. Look for meaning based on who we honestly believe the other person is today—not yesterday or pre-diagnosis.

It is wasting time and energy to get mad at each other and ourselves because one or both of us is not who we wanted them to be or who we thought they were. Wishing or faulty thinking about others only has the potential to change us. We become mad at ourselves or at the other person.

Save the energy previously devoted to self-flagellation because we have misunderstood each other, and invest it in knowing more about each other. Listen to understand, as Stephen Covey would suggest. Remember, you are only guessing as to what is right and wrong unless you first fail, as Zig Ziglar observes.

We sometimes think we are meeting each other's needs and wants when in the other person's heart and brain we are not. These are not purposeful mistakes and we should not judge ourselves. These should not be used to make ourselves feel guilty, or inadequate, or sad, or incompetent. Even in the healthiest of states, it isn't easy for human beings to understand each other. The psychological impact of the diagnosis of *dementia of the Alzheimer's type* is profound for 99.999% of the human beings who hear these words concerning themselves or a loved one. It is little wonder that communication and understanding are at best difficult between us.

Don't give up. Don't do it all your way. Don't beat yourself up for not being perfect. We're trying to deal with this old process in a brand-new and constantly changing environment.

"Whose fault is it?" is the wrong question to ask. "How can we change the process to meet existing circumstances?" is the right question!

> *We should listen to each other* as we speak today. *Take what we say, as best we can, at face value.*

P.S. When I first started to write these introspections, I promised myself I would stay away from the use of "we." W.C. Fields once said that the only people who could honestly refer to themselves as "we" were Popes (who, at certain times, claim to speak for God) and people with tapeworms.

I note and acknowledge that I am not the Pope, nor do I have a tapeworm. How, then, did this piece contain lots of "we"s? We are all human beings and subject to the same perceptual errors based on irrational thinking. (Albert Ellis was dead-on right.) However, the diseases of dementia separate the "we"s into two classes: those who make their own perceptual mistakes based on their humanness, and those who make theirs based on the diseases of dementia.

The first group comes closest to being described as "we." We have evolved to the far less than perfect state in which the human race finds itself today. The second group is often referred to as "we" and is frequently studied as "we" but is in fact not a homogeneous

group. Books on how to deal with individuals in the group are labeled as how to deal with the "we"s of dementia, but in fact we are a
group of individuals with a very, very weak "we" relationship. We all
are living with the diagnosis, but Dr. Alzheimer's impact on any one
individual, the rates at which its signs occur, and the severity of its
various effects vary significantly from person to person.

Improving understanding and communication, and knowing
and meeting each other's wants and needs, becomes a we/caregiver
and an individual/individual situation. While caregivers certainly vary
in some ways from person to person, the variation between people
living with the diseases of dementia varies as much as there are individuals with those diseases. Some physicians have told me that they
can diagnosis 85% of individuals with Alzheimer's by sitting across
the hall from them and simply observing their behaviors. Although
I personally would not like to stake a medical license on such a
method of diagnosis, all of us, to some extent, diagnose people with
Alzheimer's this way. When we expect and see stereotyped behaviors,
we turn to each other and say, "I know how they are going to act; they
have Alzheimer's disease."

The responsibility for understanding each other falls primarily
on the caregiver and, as the disease progresses, almost exclusively on
the caregiver. By the very nature of the relationship between a caregiver and the person for whom they are caring, it is the caregiver who
is best equipped to adapt to the observed changes in his or her loved
one. It is the caregiver who has more cognitive resources, better organized resources, and more consistent patterns of processing information than does the individual living with Dr. Alzheimer's sticky
size 12 bootprints in the brain.

Caregivers remain members of their "we" grouping, whereas
the persons for whom they are caring slowly become a group of one.
Some—dare I say many—healthcare professionals and experts who
pontificate about what I should do, what "we" should do, are not
(from my perspective, of course) sensitive to the fact that I am less
and less part of a "we." Caregivers are offered advice about how to
handle us "we"s, what to say to us "we"s, what "we" are thinking, and
what "we" want and need.

Unfortunately, awareness of the changes in how we understand
and communicate with each other is more and more in my caregivers'
minds, not in mine. I know this is happening to me! I seldom know,
even when it is pointed out to me, when and how the ability is in-

accessible to me. I usually believe I am still Mr. Fair, Mr. Reasonable, and Mr. Open-minded. The fact is that I am less entitled to these characterizations. I can write this. I can say this. I can believe this. The fact is, it is not true, or at least it is not as true as it was in the past. As I move from errors in judgment that I can understand with the benefit of hindsight to errors in judgment that even with the benefit of hindsight I cannot understand, so moves my ability to be a partner in this process that I have previously overdescribed!

> *I usually believe I am still Mr. Fair, Mr. Reasonable, and Mr. Open-minded. The fact is that I am less entitled to these characterizations.*

How can I know it is happening and be unable to do anything about it? How can I talk about it and still not understand or control it?

I don't know. I was hoping you could help me understand.

# If It Talks Like an It
# and Gets Lost Like an It, Is It an It?

Eighty years ago, theologian Martin Buber (1878–1965) was concerned that our society was moving from I–Thou relationships to I–It relationships. We were treating each other as if we were objects rather than human beings.

This dynamic occurs in the relationship between caregivers and individuals living with a diagnosis of Alzheimer's disease. It is happening to me.

As the weave of the lace curtain becomes thicker, as the wind blows away even the most recent of memories, people do not have time to explain to me time and again the things that I don't understand. They tire of telling me the same things over and over. They cannot depend on me to remember the simplest of instructions. My conversation is punctuated with "I forgot" and long pauses while I search for the right words. The trust relationship between husband and wife, father and son, grandfather and grandchild is breaking—not because we do not love each other as much as in the past; in fact, now our love and our connection is even more than it used to be.

> *The trust relationship between husband and wife, father and son, grandfather and grandchild is breaking—not because we do not love each other as much as in the past; in fact, now our love and our connection is even more then it used to be.*

At the same time, this stronger family connection is strained to the point of breaking by the symptoms of Alzheimer's disease.

I forget. I make promises to do some things and then I forget to do them. When reminded, I apologize, but sometimes people either get frustrated with me forgetting, or doubt that I really forgot. In either case, they know it is problematic knowing if I will now do it.

I forget that I forget. People tell me of conversations, promises, incidents which I can't recall, and I can't recall even making them—even if the details are fuzzy.

I base conclusions on incomplete and/or inaccurate memories. I inaccurately remember conversations or don't remember them at all, and then I become upset when other people seem to accuse me of making things up, or I accuse other people of not following up when, in fact, the promise to do something was all in my mind.

I act inconsistently. Previously, several times a day I told my wife I loved her. Now, some days I forget to tell her at all, and if I do tell her, I forget I've told her.

I am inconsistent in my need for repetition. I sometimes forget the same statement over and over again, or I forget it after being told just minutes ago. Sometimes I feel like a child when someone tells me something they just told me and I already knew.

In day-to-day living, I sometimes treat caregivers as "Its" and they sometimes treat me as an "It."

So, how do you relate to a Thou who does not act or think like Thou?

Inevitably, I will become an It. I will look, smell, and walk like a Thou, but I will not think and act like a Thou. It is no one's fault this happens. It just does. The Thous start lying to the It because they are tired of arguing with It. "The car has been sold"; in reality, the car is in the garage and we just don't trust It to drive. "The accountant is writing our checks"; in reality, we just do not want to argue over the fact that It cannot manage the family money. We still love Thou, but for safety and our own peace of mind we treat Thou as an It.

So, how do you relate to a Thou who does not act or think like Thou? I don't have a solution. I don't want it to happen to me. Just on my own, I don't know how to avoid it. I do know that I continue to need to be recognized as a Thou, to have my personhood recognized.

Please understand, I am still here.

# A Stranger in a Strange Land

There are times when I feel as if I am a stranger in a strange land, when the reality of the situation is that I am really myself in my own house.

It will be impossible for me to announce just when my condition has reached the point where I am unable to be a rational and equal participant in conversations about me, my behavior, and how best I should be managed for my own good and to lessen the fears of others. My family acts as if the point has come and gone, but I feel and think as if it has not yet arrived. Perhaps there is no clear line of transition from taking care of myself to being taken care of by others, but as that time approaches, I would still like to feel a part of what is going on. I would like other people to listen to me and I would like to listen to other people. I would like other people to tell me what they hear and what they feel, and I would offer them the same from me.

My caregivers always live today with fears of tomorrow. If I do this today—drive to the wrong doctor's office, forget to take the dog out for a walk, forget to close or lock the front door—isn't it just a matter of time until I do get lost and can't find my way home, forget my granddaughter is with me when I am taking a walk, forget to turn off the stove? They live and worry about tomorrow. I live and worry about *today!*

This fear and obligation of caregivers to take care of tomorrow today, before it is too late, creates situations that I am struggling to avoid. I can't argue with the logic; it is valid. I can't argue with the evidence; it inevitably happens with everyone who has Alzheimer's. But, I want the process of how we get from today to tomorrow to be open. I want to be a part of the discussions. I need updates from all observers. As it is, people indirectly update me by talking about me right in front of me or on the phone with others as if I am not even in the room. That makes me mad and sad—mad at them, and sad for us all.

Thou, yours truly, has started to become an It. Of necessity, my caregivers would argue, but nonetheless an It. The same words are used to represent me—Richard, Dad, Grandpa, my husband—but what follows does not refer to who I think and feel I am. My behavior is treated as something apart from me. "It's not him, it's the disease." Unfortunately, I am both, and to the extent the disease has altered my behavior and thinking, it has altered who I am.

I am no longer who I formerly was. I am no longer like everyone, but there is still a good deal of me left. Am I half empty or half full? What difference does it make in terms of being a full and equal member of the family? It's tough for everyone!

My heart aches and I want to shout: "I'm a different Thou, not a quarter It and three quarters Thou."

# Hello? I'm Still Here!

I have become keenly aware of a patterned response from some individuals as soon as they find out I have Alzheimer's disease. They switch their eye contact and attention to whomever I am with. It is as if knowledge of the disease immediately cloaks me in invisibility. Richard has left the room. My body may still be here, but no one who can understand what I am is at home! This happens with doctors, suit salespeople, hair cutters, produce managers, appliance repair persons, and many others.

I'm buying a suit at a department store and digging through my wallet for the card upon which I have printed all the accurate vital information I need to provide. The sales clerk notices my Alzheimer's bracelet and asks me if it is a medical alert bracelet. I say, "Yes, I have Alzheimer's disease." He turns his back to me and attempts to complete the rest of the transaction with my spouse.

I'm getting my hair cut and in the course of the conversation the stylist tells me her Dad has just been diagnosed with Alzheimer's disease. I respond, "I, too, have been diagnosed." The stylist goes into the waiting room and asks my brother to come into the salon so he can see if she is doing a good job with my haircut.

I am grocery shopping with my spouse and I am picking out Granny Smith apples and discussing with her what went on at our last Alzheimer's support meeting. The produce manager walks past us, hears the word Alzheimer's and steps between me and the Granny Smith apples and asks my wife if he can pick them out for her.

In conversation, *I* become *he*. I am gone! People also talk louder or softer, as if I am either deaf or dying. (I have always wondered why people talk more softly around ill people. Alzheimer's does not affect hearing.) You don't have to simplify your speech to make your point. You don't have to start making childlike drawings. You don't have to slow down. You don't have to *constantly* keep repeating yourself.

You do have to ask me if I understand. You do have to do more than repeat yourself. If I didn't understand it the first time around, what makes you think I will understand it the second or third time around, especially if you use the same words and just speak to me with more force and volume!?

Look me in the eyes. Make sure I am attending to what you are about to say. Don't make a speech; just tell me what you want me to know. If you have questions about if I "got" it or not, engage me in conversation and check to see if I understand. If I am having trouble understanding, use examples and comparisons with which I should be familiar. Get more of my senses involved than just words. Attribute any misunderstandings to yourself. You wrestle with trying to say it in a way I understand, but don't force me to wrestle with trying to understand what you said.

You do have to listen to me—not so that you can make me understand, but so I can understand you.

Sometimes I do and sometimes I don't understand you. Sometimes I'll tell you and sometimes I won't. I don't know why it embarrasses me when others act differently around me. I'm the one with the extra dead brain cells.

I am constantly running into memory errors, lost words, and dead ends as to what I was about to say. My internal sense of self-esteem erodes and I become defensive. Caregivers can never understand or appreciate the impact the disease has on me. They can't listen to my disjointed thought process. Because I am so unconsciously clever at covering up for my gaps, they are seldom apparent to others—just to me!

> *I don't know why it embarrasses me when others act differently around me. I'm the one with the extra dead brain cells.*

How can you support someone who sometimes feels like an It? How can you change your way of communicating with me so I can better cope with the way my listening to you is changing?

Use my name in conversation; it actually feels more affirming. Watch my face for hints that I do not understand. Sometimes I don't speak, but my nonverbals shout. Include lots of reminiscences in our conversations. I am unsure about the present, and uneasy about the future, so speaking of things I do recall is reassuring. Always look me in the eyes while speaking. Enough people have ignored me or changed their focus upon learning that I have Alzheimer's that I am extremely conscious, and self-conscious, of how people look at me when they are talking to me.

There are times when even I find it hard to find the Thou that I was before Alzheimer's.

# Christina, Mrs. Hippopotamus, and Me

Christina, my granddaughter who recently turned five years old, and I frequently end our bedtime stories with a pretend conversation between Mrs. Hippopotamus (a pink stuffed hippo who wears an old pair of Christina's pajamas) and Christina about the story we just read. As she converses with Mrs. Hippopotamus, she sometimes pauses and says, "She isn't real, right, Grandpa? You're the one who's talking?" She seems to still want to enjoy pretending, but she's old enough to check her perceptions from time to time to make sure her early childhood reality is just pretending to her five-year-old mind.

I, too, am at a stage where I sometimes am confused by fantasy (usually in the form of my own clouded recollections) and reality (usually in the form of someone else's recollections). I am moving right along in a conversation, feeling and believing it is real, and someone will say, "That's not true! That's not the way it happened! Where did you get that idea? That's not what I said."

Like Christina, I have now started to check with people to make sure that I know the difference between my own recollections (which I want to believe are always true) and the recollections of others. Unlike Christina's issue (Mrs. Hippopotamus is always me speaking), sometimes I am correct in my recollections and others are the ones who are confused and do not immediately know it. I still know this to be true, at least once in a while.

Others who know I have Alzheimer's generally assume that they are correct and that my disease causes me to be incorrect. When my recollections are corrected based on the generalization that my disease guarantees I am wrong, I lose another ounce of self-confidence in my ability to know and remember what is going on around me. This is still, and in fact more and more, important to me.

> *When my recollections are corrected based on the generalization that my disease guarantees I am wrong, I lose another ounce of self-confidence.*

Please accentuate the positive with my recollections. Don't lie if I'm not accurate, but don't try to make me remember exactly like you do. About some things, I'm more accurate than you, and remember that my ability to recall accurately is more important to me than yours is to you.

---

This is the "plan" I adopted to help Christina improve her reading:

Learning to read is hard work for children. Read books with rhymes. Teach your child rhymes, short poems, and songs. Play simple word games. Help your child separate the sounds in words, listen for beginning and ending sounds, and put separate sounds together. Point out the letter–sound relationships your child is learning on labels, boxes, newspapers, magazines and signs. Listen to your child read words and books from school. Be patient and listen as your child practices. Let your child know you are proud of his or her reading. Make reading a part of every day. Read together every day. Spend time talking about stories, pictures, and words.

*http://www.nifl.gov/partnershipforreading/publications/html/parent_broch/*

# Muddled Puddles

From time to time, spouses, parents, friends, and children stumble through puddles and inadvertently splash water on themselves and each other, causing all parties to become upset. Usually, over time, the water dries, leaving only faint outlines on clothing and no marks on the skin. Alzheimer's disease seems to muddle these puddles. It seems to add an ingredient to the puddles that changes their nature.

When caregivers stumble through puddles, they are left with stains on their clothing and on their skin. When people with Alzheimer's stumble through the puddle, they are left with holes in their clothes which only they can see, and a stinging, burning sensation on their skin, which only they can feel.

Prior to my diagnosis, I stumbled from time to time. I forgot to do this or that. I said something that was true but I said it in an insensitive or inappropriate manner. I argued with my wife. I stumbled when dealing with others.

Now, when I forget, people tell me it is okay because it is the disease, not me.

Now when I make a mistake, people tell me it's the disease's fault, not mine.

When I blurt out something I would like to take back and swallow, people tell me that inappropriate outbursts simply come with the disease. When others tell me it is not my fault and attribute it to the disease, it leaves the stain of Alzheimer's on their clothing and skin, and a sharp burning sensation in my mind.

Prior to my diagnosis, my wife and I stumbled from time to time. We argued about inconsequential things: where we should eat, who spends more money on unnecessary clothes, where we should place the Christmas tree. These issues seemed to resolve themselves. Now when we argue, we both start out from the assumption that one person will not understand the other. I have the disease, and my wife has her fears that color her perceptions of everything. We are left stained and stinging, even by small, inconsequential puddles.

Prior to the diagnosis, I stumbled with others from time to time. I was sometimes a tad arrogant. I was also funny, clever, and usually very kind. Others were willing to overlook my drive. After all, I was frequently right! Now, I am characterized by others as sometimes out of control. "The disease has changed you," they tell me. "You aren't the person you used to be." I am burning and have no ointment to put on my oozing, bright-red, first- and second-degree burns.

I react to puddles that never seemed to bother me before Dr. Alzheimer's discovery found its way into my brain. Others react to puddles that didn't seem to bother them before Dr. Alzheimer's discovery found its way into my brain.

Who cared if I got a traffic ticket? Who cared if I got lost going to someplace new? Who cared if I messed up a meal because I forgot a key ingredient? Who really cared if I didn't close the front door all the way? If my family didn't know where I was for a couple of hours, no one was concerned.

Who cares now? Everyone!

People accuse me of being paranoid, when in fact I'm only responding to the sting of puddles that are invisible or inconsequential to them. I can see the puddles, but they sometimes can't. I feel them, but they can't. For a while, I thought they saw them but simply would not acknowledge them.

What I have come to realize is that others can't be with me between my ears (only Mr. Spock can mind-meld), and so they are unaware of the new puddles I splash through

*People continually tell me, "You don't look or sound like you have Alzheimer's. I see you as the same Richard I have always seen."*

hundreds of times a day. These puddles weren't there before the tsunami of forgetfulness cascaded through my brain, caused by the frequent quakes of Alzheimer's disease.

People continually tell me, "You don't look or sound like you have Alzheimer's. I see you as the same Richard I have always seen."

But don't you know? I didn't understand this, I misunderstood that. I couldn't remember this. I mistakenly did that. All of these "this or that's" are initially cognitive activities before they become observable behaviors.

Bright people, I am told, are better at unconsciously and consciously hiding the consequences of their Alzheimer's from others. Too bad for everyone I was once real bright.

# A Distinction Without a Difference

✕✦✕✦✕✦✕✦✕

*"When I use a word," Humpty Dumpty said, in rather*
*a scornful tone, "it means just what I choose*
*it to mean—neither more nor less."*
*"The question is," said Alice, "whether you can make*
*words mean so many different things."*
*"The question is," said Humpty Dumpty, "which is to*
*be master—that's all."*
—http://www.sabian.org/Alice/lgchap06.htm

Words not only describe my world, they create my world. What happens when the meaning of words changes from one day to the other, from one hour to the other, or when words sometimes lose their meaning? This is where I and my world are right now.

As my short-term memory dissolves and I can only recall bits and pieces of conversations, I find myself arguing with caregivers about the exact words that were used. Unfortunately, I am now discovering that the words don't matter because we are each interpreting the meanings through our own filters. They are arguing as if I were one of them, because there, in their world, is where they want to keep me. There is where they want to believe I am. There is where they see and hear me.

I am arguing from where I am: with gaps in my recollections, with misunderstandings as to what was said first and what was said second, with blank spaces in their words and world. Yes, I still have the need to remain someone who I am not—one of them—who I was, not who I am!

I say, "I want to buy a dog the day after our present dog dies."

My wife, and in fact my entire family, replies, "You can't take care of a dog. We don't want the additional responsibility of taking care of a dog and you. Dogs pee on the wood floors, leave hair all over, and are an unwanted additional concern when left alone because we want to go visit someone. And besides, why are we talking about this? You already have a dog who is alive."

I say, "All dogs pee; I can't be held responsible for accidents. I clean the house. There is nowhere I want to go. Don't you understand I need a dog, a big dog?"

They respond, "We don't want another dog. All dogs pee, and have accidents, and we can't trust you to take the dog out enough to keep them from messing up the house. Can't you understand why we don't want another dog?"

I respond, "Can't you understand why I want another dog?"

What they *intended* to communicate was, "We already feel inadequate and overwhelmed taking care of you. Give us a break, and when there is an opportunity for us to have less responsibility, let us have it. Please. Especially if it only means not having a dog."

What I *intended* to communicate was, "I am already feeling insecure and lonely. The thought of not having another dog giving me unconditional love when all that I need to do is provide two cups of food a day, some ear rubbing, and a daily long walk makes me even more frightened of the future."

I tried to debate them point by point, but I forgot some of their points and misunderstood others. Neither of us really thought the issue through; they were forced to jump into it when I up and announced I was getting another dog when Annie died. They jumped in with a bunch of words, and I responded with a bunch of words. The real distinctions between us were never spoken.

Neither side affirmed the feelings of the other.

It was a debate, plain and simple. The winner was the one who did the better job of debating. I *thought* I'd won. I don't think I'll get another dog when Annie dies.

> *Would a dictionary resolve our misunderstandings? Would a tape recorder resolve our lack of clear communication? No!*

Lots of words were exchanged, but the distinctions between my caregivers and me were not addressed or resolved.

Thanks to my brother (who was not present at the dog fight) for reviewing and explaining this to me.

The distinctions on which we focus are rhetorically and grammatically real. Would a dictionary resolve our misunderstandings?

Would a tape recorder resolve our lack of clear communication? No! For me, their distinctions, their differences, don't have meaning.

Why can't they understand that? Why can't they understand me?

There is both no answer and many answers to this hard question. The larger and more important the issue, the more we seem to avoid it and concentrate on the details. My hope is that we can all try harder to communicate with less emphasis on nouns, verbs, dictionary meanings, who said what, and when did they say it, and more on the *feeling* meaning of what we are trying to tell each other.

---

Wanna see the impact of words on other other words, on meaning, and on your feelings?

Welcome to Crazy Libs! Read brief stories with your words strategically inserted to produce wacky results. Original stories, excerpts from classic literature, and excerpts from elsewhere on the RinkWorks site are featured. It's silly nonsense fun every time.

*http://rinkworks.com/crazylibs/*

# "Play It Again, Caregivers"

*Rick:* You know what I want to hear.
*Sam:* [lying] No, I don't.
*Rick:* You played it for her, you can play it for me!
*Sam:* [lying] Well, I don't think I can remember . . .
*Rick:* If she can stand it, I can! Play it!

—Casablanca (1942)

Many Christmases ago, my wife gave me a coffee cup on which was inscribed the words, *It is not that I don't hear and understand what you said, it's that I don't believe you.* That was an eye-opener for me. I always assumed that people who didn't do what I asked them to do simply didn't hear me. It never dawned on me that they didn't want to do it or, worse yet, didn't believe it was necessary to do.

> *It is not that I don't hear and understand what you said, it's that I don't believe you.*

The shoe is now on the other foot. My family will ask me to do something, and I don't do it. Early in the disease process, they assumed I didn't hear them. They would tell me again. This got old after a while. They became annoyed at having to tell me the same thing over and over again. Later on, they realized there was a possibility that my twisted brain fibers actually didn't understand their words. They felt appropriately guilty.

Their current dilemma continues to be to figure out just why I am not complying with their requests. Is it because it hasn't registered in my brain? Is it because I can't figure it out? Is it because I forgot it? Is it because I don't believe them? Is it because I don't want to do it?

Old strategies that worked for years—say it again and say it louder—just don't work any more. I'm glad I'm not a caregiver who has to figure me out every day.

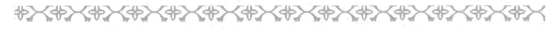

## INSIGHTS FOR FAMILIES
## COPING WITH ALZHEIMER'S DISEASE

- Allow your loved one with Alzheimer's disease to express herself verbally and creatively.

- Advocate for autonomy, choice, and independence. Don't always jump in and try to help your loved one. Let him do it himself.

- Create a healthy habitat, environment, and atmosphere.

- Encourage discussion of present and future. Don't only reminisce.

- Your loved one may have greater fear and concern with "looking stupid" or being embarrassed in public than in forgetting things.

- You will likely have to rearrange your lifestyle, perhaps retiring early or moving.

- Explore and implement legal and financial planning changes as soon after diagnosis as possible after consulting skilled professionals.

*http://www.healingwell.com/library/alzheimers/bryce1.asp*

# My Champion or My Hero?

*Because I do love you, I give to you my life, my dreams and all of my tomorrows. I promise to cherish you through good and bad times. In sickness and in health, I'll care. I'll laugh with you. I'll cry with you. I promise I will do my share to keep our marriage ever new. I'll live with you, I'll grow with you. I'll work to make the life we share as beautiful, as sweet and rare, as the love I feel today for you.*

—Linda's wedding vow to Richard

I realize I haven't written a lot about my caregivers. I am clear about much of the dynamics and impact this disease is having on me, but I am unclear about how this is affecting my caregivers. I have shared my life with them and they with me. We have created a life together, different than it would have been apart. The expectations we had worked out together don't seem to work as they did in the past. We all still look and sound the same, but I am different and so, too, are they.

I love them. I have lived with them for many, many years. Some of them I have raised. The leader of my caregiver team is my spouse, Linda. As she doesn't always seem to understand me, it is also increasingly difficult for me to always understand her (not that I was a master at it pre-Alzheimer's!). We look the same as we did in our last anniversary picture. I know I don't think the same, and neither of us thinks about each other the same way as we did when we took that picture.

Real or imagined personality changes, thinking patterns, and fears growing out of the Alzheimer's diagnosis have shuffled our own cards, and our couple's cards, and our family's deck. Alzheimer's is changing how I think and what she and I think of ourselves, each other, and us. Before we married, I saw my wife's strength of personality as an attractive attribute. For years since then, I devoted a good deal of my time to resisting that strength. I now have an appreciation and admiration for how she uses that strength to support me, to protect me, to nurture me in ways neither of us thought would ever be necessary.

I am a big guy, and I was a very smart guy; I never thought of myself as needing protection. But I do. I need to be protected from myself and my increasingly frequent misperceptions of what's going on around me. I need to be supported because my self-esteem and self-confidence, which once served as a major attraction for my spouse, are turning into self-doubt and hesitancy.

Old age reverses our evolution of independence from childhood. We become more dependent on others to do things for us. Alzheimer's quickens this evolutionary reversal and adds many idiosyncratic twists to the process. It's slightly different for everyone, but its effect is the same: We become unable to take care of ourselves.

*Many times, she must guess when I need help and when I don't. Asking for help does not come easy for me. If she guesses wrong, I am not pleased. If she guesses right, I sometimes take it for granted.*

I'm not sure if Linda is my champion or my hero. Heroes are usually shared with others. Champions are more personal. Heroes are worshiped from afar. Champions generally embrace the values and feelings of those they champion. With heroes, it's usually the other way around. I think she is more my personal champion than my hero. It is a wonderful feeling to know I have a champion. I feel more secure in myself, in my future, and in our future knowing she is there—shield in one hand and lance in the other. What was an attraction, and then an annoyance, has again become an attraction! More and more I depend on her constancy, her strength, her sense of purpose, her self-assurance.

Being my champion involves much, much more than remembering to tell me to take my pills. It's being a best friend, lover, appointment secretary, OnStar advisor, personal cheerleader, constant optimist, financial manager, driver, housekeeper, groundskeeper, handy-woman, and cook, and meeting any and all of my other occasional spoken and unspoken personal needs. *Where are my glasses? What day is it? Where are we going? Tell me again.* Many times, she must guess when I need help and when I don't. Asking for help does not come easy for me. If she guesses wrong, I am not pleased. If she guesses right, I sometimes take it for granted.

My spouse has wrapped herself around me, providing enough space for me to sometimes stumble around by my own stubborn self, but not to fall and hurt myself. She is my spokeswoman and buffer from those who don't understand. She is my advocate with professionals who sometimes are too busy to give me the attention and support I need. She has always been my best friend, yet now she is there for me in ways neither of us ever imagined. We have always treated each other as equals and operated from the principle that one plus one equals three. Right now it feels like one plus me equals about one and three-fourths. I know I am not pulling my own weight. I am pulling her down. She sometimes pulls just for me and sometimes for both of us. Every morning she absorbs the cares of yesterday and willingly faces the increasing cares of today. Every day I see that I can pull less and less. I know this must be wearing her down.

Like it or not, I am increasingly dependent on my champion to figure it out for me. I am depending on my champion to figure it out all by herself. I am depending on my champion to figure it out for the two of us. Daily, more and more of my independence is morphing into dependence on Linda.

Thank you, Linda, for thousands of yesterdays, today, and as many tomorrows as drugs, my love for you, and my will and your love for me will create for me and for us.

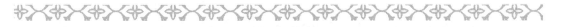

## WHO PROVIDES ALZHEIMER'S CARE?

More than 7 out of 10 people with Alzheimer's disease live at home, where almost 75% of their care is provided by family and friends. The remainder is "paid" care costing an average of $19,000 per year. Families pay almost all of that out of pocket.

Half of all nursing home residents have Alzheimer's disease or a related disorder.

*http://www.alz.org/AboutAD/statistics.asp*

# Once Again, My Children Believe They Know More Than I Do

✕✦✕✦✕✦✕✦✕

Every parent goes through the stage, whether or not he or she wants to: The child is convinced he or she is cursed with the dumbest parents in the world. The stage usually starts when the child is 11 or 12 years old and ends when the child is 19, 21, 28, or 32—although I have read of cases from distant lands where children reached their mid-60s before realizing their parents were not "stupid."

My children went through that stage. Usually, the argument ended with a frustrated me saying, "Because I'm your father and I said so!" When my son was 22, he sent his mother an "I'm so sorry for the way I treated you two" note. She still carries it around in her purse!

Unfortunately, my kids are starting to act that way again. They isolate me from their day-to-day lives. They do not want to hear what I have to say about most anything. When I walk into a room, they abruptly stop talking to each other. When I come across my spouse on the phone to one of them, she looks guilty and starts talking in obvious code. She uses one-word answers and says, "I can't say right now" a lot. It is very difficult to live in a situation where my five-year-old granddaughter honestly believes I am one of the smartest people in the world because I am a former teacher and she has yet to ask me a question I did not know the answer to. On the other hand, the adults seldom ask me any questions and never ask me to help them with their home/work. When I do offer unsolicited advice, they are most likely to respond with a disinterested "Thanks, but I'll take care of it myself." I never claimed to know it all, but I still know some thing(s)! I have not forgotten 62 years of my life experience. I went to school for almost 20 years of my life. (I now know it was way, way too long to spend worrying about how to read and write, add and subtract, and do unto others as I would have others do unto me—but hey, I didn't make the rules for granting degrees. Someone should come up with a child's edition of Stephen Covey's *7 Habits of Highly Effective People* and after children have memorized them they should be free to quit school whenever they feel bored, and return to school whenever they feel bored.) I must have learned some one thing of value in all those years that they don't know and that may some time in the course of their lives be of some value to them.

My kids used to ask me if I would or could; they said "please" and "thank you" to me. They would never think of raising their voices when addressing me; now they tell me what I may and may not do. Formerly, when I asked them a direct question, I expected and got a direct answer. Now when I ask, they answer, "We'll see. I have to think about it. I do not want to talk about that right now." My way of dealing with this is to try to ignore it. "No, that's it, end of discussion. You are the one with Alzheimer's and sometimes we have to make the decision without your input and it's already been made." Responses like this always hurt. I feel sad sometimes and mad other times.

Although they are not always the most tactful of individuals, they are trying their best. They don't know how to respond to me, just as I don't know how to deal with them. Sometimes we just have to deal with each other as is. I try to anticipate clash points, make it easier to all concerned by suggesting solutions before there is a point of contention that causes them to band together and react as a group. I offered to stop driving. I asked that the finances be managed by someone other than yours truly. An unanticipated consequence of my anticipatory actions was they were upset with me for prematurely making these decisions and forcing them to do some things (drive me to appointments, balance the checkbook, etc.) that they thought they should not have to do quite yet.

Obviously, there are no "right answers" and no "right ways." Most families, like ours, keep trying until we get it approximately right and hope we have not alienated each other in the process.

I believe that the best strategy to avoid inadvertently hurting each others' feelings or offending each other is to keep talking. It seems as if we only talk openly about the disease and ourselves when there is a decision to be made or announced. We are all tired of talking about Alzheimer's disease. We are all tired of talking about me as if I were an old family pet who is increasingly a burden to all but still beloved by all. One who has its good

> *Obviously, there are no "right answers" and no "right ways." Most families, like ours, keep trying until we get it approximately right and hope we have not alienated each other in the process.*

days and bad days and has become erratic in its behavior. Everyone still wants it around, but since it isn't acting like it formerly did, folks seem a little short tempered with when it doesn't behave.

I know I am not thought of as the family pet, nor do I feel like I am the family pet. But I also know that I am not perceived the same way as I was before we were told, "He has dementia, probably of the Alzheimer's type."

Yes, sometimes my children do know more and better than do I, but I still know some things. Trying to decide where to draw the independence line is easier said than done. The problem is that we are not saying enough. When we do not talk enough prior to drawing lines, they are always, in my opinion, drawn wrong. Present circumstances require us to talk more, not less. Even though it is no guarantee of success, if we do not try we are guaranteed, at best, limited success and, at worst, hurt feelings, which can lead to failure. Not talking most often leads to blaming and name calling and ensures that no one will talk with me the next time before it is necessary to make a decision.

Somehow, it worked better for me when I said, "Because I'm your father." I am still their father, but I am not the person I was. And everyone knows it, but no one seems to know what to do about it.

# Sex, Side Effects, Alzheimer's, and Intimacy

When I was diagnosed, the neurologist volunteered the information that Alzheimer's would not affect my sex life. In fact, he told me, "Sometimes you will have sex, roll over and forget you just had it, and then want to have it again." "Wow!" I thought. "There might be an up side to Alzheimer's—*more sex!*"

How stupid of me to regress back to my late teens and 20s and focus on quantity of sex and exclude consideration of the real issue: intimacy between spouse, family, and friends.

For me, more or less, better or worse sex is a secondary effect of one of the major influences this disease has had on me. (I put the word *sex* in the title so everyone would want to read this!) In my distant past, once I found out that sex was not enough to create or maintain an intimate relationship, I began exploring additional components to create and maintain intimate relationships. There are levels within levels of intimacy. There are physical levels, emotional levels, intellectual levels, and levels of shared activities. The operational definition of precisely what constitutes intimacy changes with age, circumstances, and experience, but for me, prior to the diagnosis, I was at least moving in the right direction! I was trying to deepen the relationships with my spouse, with my family, and with friends (each, of course, defined by different behaviors) to the levels at which each of us would feel comfortable characterizing them as intimate.

Alzheimer's disease shuffles the intimacy deck! It upsets the apple cart. It's a whole new ball game.

Alzheimer's disease creates opportunities both to expand intimacy and to pull away from intimacy. And I thought that after 40 years of wrestling with those issues, I had finally overcome them. Along comes a magnifying glass called Alzheimer's, and I'm right back into them.

My relationship with my spouse, my family, and my friends has broadened and in some ways deepened. We spend more time really being together. We talk more, we hug more, we cry more, we laugh more and harder and longer together.

In other ways I have pulled back into myself and pushed them away—sending mixed messages. I am subject to quicker changes in my moods. I get angrier, it happens more often, and it happens quicker. I say things that others take in ways I didn't mean or intend. I, the "great communicator," search for words and frequently substitute long, rambling explanations and examples in place of saying what I mean. They didn't ask for this. They don't deserve it. I just do it! It happens every day, mostly in ways I am not aware of until the harm has been done.

> *We spend more time really being together. We talk more, we hug more, we cry more, we laugh more and harder and longer together.*

The diagnosis has a side effect that is not listed in any of the drug pamphlets. It is fear! We all live with fear: spouses, family members, friends, and of course yours truly. Fear has contaminated our hearts, minds, and feelings. It's worse than cancer because we can't cut it out. We can't kill it with radiation. We cry, we get mad, we get sad, and we get scared—all as a result of the fear that courses through our bodies.

I am frequently suspect of individuals who profess to have been born again in a very positive sense by the disease, i.e., "The flowers smell sweeter, the sun shines brighter, I love everyone more." For me, at least, the disease swings a double-edged sword. It cuts through barriers and provides opportunities for more intimacy, for deeper intimacy, while at the same time the fact that it is cutting through my brain, cutting short my life span, and cutting out my memory creates a poison in me. This poison has yet to be purged by the possibilities, the positive possibilities, this diagnosis presents to me. I simply have not devised a strategy to keep fears, real and imagined, from poisoning intimacy.

I struggle with this every day. Those around me struggle with mine and their own struggles every day.

Many years ago, a good day, a great weekend, was closely correlated with the amount and quality of sex (mostly amount). As I became older, quality was more important than quantity. As I became still older, I was finally able to place sex as a part of intimacy rather than vice versa. There are no pills that increase or decrease my ability to be intimate. I can't blame Prozac. I can't rely on Viagra. There is no pill to help me maintain or expand my intimacy with my spouse, my family, and my friends.

I believe that my fears, which I of course blame on Dr. Alzheimer, are my real enemies. They are the cause of my intimacy issues. But in the end, who causes my fears? What causes my fears? What intensifies and controls my fears? Plaques in my brain? A deteriorating hippocampus? Inflammation in my frontal lobe? All of the above? These are questions for the psychologists and the neurologists to answer. What I, Richard Taylor, owner of a rapidly evolving personality and a slowly failing memory, must deal with is myself.

---

Emotional intimacy is a dimension of interpersonal intimacy which varies in degree, much like physical intimacy. In an emotional context, intimacy can be observed in terms of communication pertaining to emotional states as subjective experiences. The degree of comfort and effectiveness of the communicative process can be seen as an indicator of the emotional intimacy between two individuals. Relative emotional intimacy depends primarily on trust, as well as the nature of the relationship. Emotional intimacy frequently involves individuals discussing their feelings and emotions with each other in order to gain understanding and offer mutual support. It is necessary for human beings to have this form of intimacy on a regular basis for them to develop and maintain good mental health.

*http://en.wikipedia.org/wiki/Emotional_intimacy*

---

# Hanging On with My Tongue

I'm not sure what family and friends expect to hear when they begin a conversation with me. But I do know that somewhere near the end of the conversation, many of them say to me, "I just can't believe you have Alzheimer's." The reason they offer why they can't believe I have Alzheimer's is because "You sound and look like the same old Richard."

I do still speak in complete sentences. Most of the time I am able to stay on-topic. I am still, from time to time, an entertaining speaker. I can still recall and frequently use many of the words in *30 Days to a More Powerful Vocabulary*.

Fortunately for me, my conversation partners have yet to perceive my need to direct the conversation. If I am interrupted, or asked a question, the response may not be appropriate or I may avoid answering the question. If I am interrupted, I may not come back to where I was before the interruption. Is it my own vanity or shame, or fear or low self-esteem that keeps me from asking for prompts or help?

Sometimes I do not respond directly to the other end of a conversation because I can't find the information within myself to form my response. When I attempt to participate in a discussion with more than one other person, I am either the leader of the discussion or an observer commenting on what has been said. Sometimes I even offer powerful and insightful responses, but unfortunately and increasingly frequently they are four or five sentences behind where they should have been interjected. It usually stops the conversation as people pause to try and politely figure out what I am talking about. I now spend lots more time searching for the right word: "You know what I'm talking about. It's like . . . You know what I mean."

> *Sometimes I do not respond directly to the other end of a conversation because I can't find the information within myself to form my response.*

Just recently, I have noticed that I have to search for a complete thought, not just a word or two.

I still sound and look like Richard. My one-on-one conversations sound pretty much like they always sounded. My internal conversations are another matter. Sometimes I just want to shout at others: "I'm having trouble—you don't know it, and I don't know how to ask for help with this problem!"

I am now fully engaged in a battle to maintain, access, and control my thoughts and mind. I know I will eventually have to gulp and surrender.

Serious depression develops in more than 20% of people with Alzheimer's disease, and in up to 50% of Alzheimer's caregivers. Most people never get help for this treatable illness.

*http://www.alz.org/Health/Counseling/depression.asp*

# A Silent, One-Sided
# Conversation with My Caregivers

Like the teacher in the comic strip *Peanuts*—whose students only understand her to be saying "Wah wah, wah, wah," when in fact she is attempting to teach and explain the world—I speak to my caregivers and they seem to understand every word, every thought. Yet they do not behave as if they have heard me.

I'm mad.

I'm sad.

I'm scared.

I'm worried for me and for you.

I'm worried I don't have enough resources to get me through this.

I'm worried I am the cause of the impact this disease is having and will have on you.

I'm worried you keep telling me "not to worry about anything, I will take care of you."

I'm worried that I'm not worth it.

I'm worried your love for the "former" me will be replaced with a resigned acceptance of the "new" me.

I'm worried things won't be like we planned and hoped.

I'm worried because I am less sure than usual who I am, and who I will be.

I'm worried I can't help you, and you believe you can help me.

I'm worried you might be right; perhaps you "can't do this."

I'm worried because I'm not the pillar of strength, the font of wisdom, the shoulder to cry on that I thought I was (even though in fact I knew that was an exaggerated self-image).

I'm worried you will need other shoulders to support you.

I'm worried your love will wear thin and commitment will begin to replace love.

I'm worried commitment will wear thin and obligation will begin to replace commitment.

I'm very worried and even more frustrated . . .

# Religion, Spirituality, Alzheimer's, and Richard

I have visited a few Alzheimer's care facilities, and all of them offer voluntary Sunday services. This is usually a nondenominational Christian service, and occasionally a Jewish service on Saturday. "Guests" are walked, wheeled, and encouraged to get out of their rooms and come to the community room. They sing a few hymns, usually accompanied by some group from a local church, sit through a reading from the Bible and 5–15 minutes of a message with a religious theme, and then depart to the lunchroom for lunch. In some facilities, guests are encouraged to sit outside and enjoy the weather, the sun, the day, the moment.

Journals and convention panels increasingly are exploring the need and the most appropriate ways to address the spiritual concerns of individuals with Alzheimer's disease. Physicians are encouraged to consider the impact of the illness on spirit and soul as a part of their treatment plans. Prayers, chants, and readings are created and collected especially for individuals with Alzheimer's disease.

Many people have asked me if I feel more spiritual since I was diagnosed, more in touch with my own spirituality. As my mind clears itself of memories, am I closer to my soul? To God? To the life forces within and around me?

Thus far, I can confidently report no more or less spiritual insights into the creation, the creator, or myself. I do not feel closer, farther away, more or less in touch—period. I do have the distinct sense I am withdrawing from living, and nothing seems waiting to rush in to fill the void I already feel.

It seems an assumption of society that as individuals grow older, the need to feel closer to or the sense of being a part of something larger than themselves, or the belief that there is some thing or place waiting to welcome them after death, should be and is increasingly important to them. After all, aren't there a disproportionately large number of "old" people in our churches? Isn't our grandmother the only one in the family who sings hymns and talks about God? What about all those deathbed conversions?

If this need grows within us as we age, shouldn't a disease that produces behaviors associated with growing older increase the need, even within 30- and 40-year-old early-onset individuals, to tend to spiritual needs? Isn't it then in the best interests of the "patient" to begin to look for and treat symptoms of a need for religion or spirituality?

I realize these are gross generalizations. My intention is not to offer a sociological or psychological analysis of the role of religion in our society or in the treatment and support of individuals with Alzheimer's disease. My purpose is to try and understand why caregivers seem intent on introducing, reinforcing, or just plain imposing values, beliefs, and religious practices on people they love and respect—the individual with Alzheimer's disease whom they have devoted a large part of their lives to taking care of.

There is also the larger issue of caregivers meeting their own wants and needs through interpretation of the behaviors of the individual for whom they care. Spirituality is one of the major vehicles used to deliver hope to the caregivers. Hope that their loved one is still with them. Hope that their loved one is at peace with them. Hope that there is still a shared set of values that connects their loved one with them.

If I was an active member of a religious organization prior to Stage 2 or 3, there is no reason to end my participation (at whatever level that might be) when I move into end-stage. However, if religion was not a real focus of my life, why should caregivers decide for me that as the shadow of death comes over me I should convert, or "act" religious? If what is happening to me has influenced the beliefs of my caregivers, and they feel the need for more religious ritual and activity, why take me along for the ride (in my theoretical wheelchair) simply because I cannot comment on what is happening? As I understand most organized religions, you cannot be saved or improved unless you do it yourself and believe it yourself. While I do not question your intentions to do what is best for me, isn't this primarily best for you?

Physicians, friends, and family are forever asking me, "How is it going? Do you still feel okay? Having any problems?" The measures used to evaluate my answers seem to grow from the unstated question, "Are you still like me?" On many occasions, I have watched caregivers read into even the smallest of reflex responses: "See, he still knows me." I have heard psychologists and physicians reassuringly say, "We really don't know exactly what that means, but it could be she [fill in a positive and supportive interpretation of even the small-est of behaviors]."

The need for my caregivers to feel connected to the "old" me rather than the "now" me is understandable, even long after I have lost the need to reciprocate. However, I must say this: I hope you would honor in the same way my need for dignity when I cannot re-spond to you as when I could. Please treat me first as a human being, and then as the loving person I once was. Of course, if I do not know what is going on around me, why should I care what you are doing to me or with me? That is a good question, and probably speaks to my own needs to try to control what is happening to me long after I have lost the interest or ability to do so. This stuff is not easy to figure out before it happens, you know.

Once I stop talking; once I lose control over my capacity to use sound to form words that are symbols representing my thoughts; once I stoop over in my chair, never to rise again by myself or express what I know and feel, will I be aware of what has happened to me? I may still be able to offer a responsive blink or a tapping toe, but these responses are in response to your framing of a question and no one knows if I have the capacity to understand what you are asking. We are probably both guessing: you for the best interpretation, and I for . . . we will never know.

Measure my brain waves; speculate on the patterns in relation-ship to the presented stimulus. What do they mean to me? Unfortu-nately, caregivers are forced to guess. Educated and idiosyncratic as these guesses are, please remember this isn't me, it is you guessing for me (and/or for you). If you can't know if I am hot or cold, or both, or neither, how will you know if my spirit is strong or weak? You cannot know for sure if I am looking forward to death and a life-after-death experience, or if I want or need to attend Sunday services.

> *If you can't know if I am hot or cold, or both, or neither, how will you know if my spirit is strong or weak?*

For the moment, I don't sense a grow-ing need to change what I believe and feel about life after death, baptism, the first or the second coming, and the rest of the Apostles' or Nicene Creed. I do have a somewhat different insight into my concept of and feelings about spirit and spirituality, but it seems to have nothing to do with religion, at least as I understand it.

Written by an individual born without arms or legs:

    Too often we underestimate the power of a touch, a smile, a kind word, a listening ear, an honest compliment, or the smallest act of caring, all of which have the potential to turn a life around. People come into our lives for a reason, a season, or a lifetime. Embrace all equally.

*http://ajitchouhan.blogspot.com/2006/05/human-spirit.html*

# Plants as Pets

Who or what makes the best companion for someone with Alzheimer's disease? A dog, a cat, a bird, a hamster, or some other furry little animal? What about the TV, the VCR, the DVD player? Let's not forget the chair by the window, or the bed. Of course, there is always Ambien, melatonin, or a bottle of Richard's Wild Irish Rose.

How should you select a pet for yourself or your loved one? Is the pet inexpensive? Can the pet easily be replaced with almost an exact look-alike? Can you grow the pet yourself and watch it evolve from a seedling to an infant to an adult? Can you cut off one part of the pet and grow a companion without having to go to South Korea to have it cloned?

Other than an eager member of the opposite sex (who can provide warmth, comfort, and joy both in and out of bed and in ways which if attempted with an animal would be deemed socially inappropriate), I would like to suggest that plants make the best pets. They can remind us of the past or the present. They smell good all the time (we have more brain cells devoted to smell than any other sense). They don't poop, ever. You need never take them out for a walk; you can just move them from window to window. They grow fast and, given some imagination, they develop personalities. As a bonus, you can assign their gender and they will not mind.

Actually, what I need is to feel that I am still taking care of something. Something that returns love, that gives itself away without expecting anything back, that wants to please me . . . all the time! Something that never, ever judges me but just accepts me for who and what I am at that particular moment. Something that is not hung-up about who I was, or who I am, or who I will be. Something that is more concerned with getting water and food for today, rather

> . . . what I need is to feel that I am still taking care of something. . . . Something that never, ever judges me but just accepts me for who and what I am at that particular moment.

than worrying whether I'll be around in five or six years. Something that is happy to be with me no matter where I live, or am forced to live (for my own good, of course). Something that remembers little or nothing of yesterday, but does its best to make today the best day of its life and, quite unintentionally, the best day of my life.

I vote for plants!

# Give Me Your
# Money, Your Car, and . . .

I can't imagine how difficult it is for a spouse to have to say to a partner, for a child to say to his or her mom or dad or to a sister or brother, "I'll take care of the money and your car, and I'll take you when and where you need to go."

I do know what it feels like for a person (me) to have that said to him by his spouse. It was dramatic and traumatic for both of us. Both of us see it as something that must be done.

"It's in your interest," says my spouse.

"No, it's in *your* best interest," I say to my spouse.

"But I am in a better position to make this judgment than you," says my spouse.

"I am still competent to make this decision," I say to my spouse.

"Our kids think this is best for you," says my spouse. "The doctor thinks it's best," says my spouse. "If you don't do it, then the police or the courts will have to do it," says my spouse. "And, oh, by the way, stop feeling so paranoid; everyone is not out to get you," says my spouse.

*Give me all your money.*

I have always sympathized with children who have no access to money of their own, and whose spending is wholly dependent on the whims of adults. Children watch adults spend money in ways that in a child's mind, I'm sure, seem frivolous. Kids hear adults say, "We don't have the money," and then go out and buy adult toys, whatever they may be, which are of no value or use to a child. They hear their parents say, "You can't understand what it's like to be responsible for raising you. You can't understand what it's like to work for a living. You can't understand what it's like to be responsible for the financial future of another human being. I am the only one working and I have to pay all the bills."

I now completely understand what a child feels like.

> *"And, oh, by the way, stop feeling so paranoid; everyone is not out to get you."*

*Give me your car.*

I know what it's like to walk out to my garage and get in my car and turn the key and the car won't start. My whole life comes to a stop: I can't go anywhere, and I'm stuck here. I get on the phone and start rearranging my life and put it basically on hold until I can have someone come out and fix my car. I have the sense of being trapped in my house. All the plans I had made for the day and perhaps for the week come to a crashing halt. I simply can't get there. I can't get anywhere.

Don't you understand? I feel trapped in my own house!

I *am* trapped in my own house!

All the people I wanted to see, all the things I wanted to do, all the errands I wanted to run are put on hold. My car won't start. I become restless when the repair person is late coming out. I try to fix the car myself, to no avail. I try to borrow my neighbor's car. I try to call a cab.

It's no use, I'm stuck.

Now that I am living with Alzheimer's disease, here I sit at home.

My car starts; it works.

I do neither. I'm stuck. I'm trapped in a broken mind in my own house!

# PREVENTION MEASURES FOR WANDERING

- Encourage movement and exercise to reduce anxiety, agitation, and restlessness.

- Ensure that all basic needs are met (e.g., toileting, nutrition, thirst).

- Involve the person in daily activities such as folding laundry or preparing dinner.

- Place color-matching cloth over doorknobs to camouflage.

- Redirect pacing or restless behavior.

- Place a mirror near doorways. The reflection of a person's own face will often stop him or her from exiting the door.

- Reassure the person if he or she feels lost, abandoned, or disoriented.

- Inform your neighbors and local emergency responders of the person's condition and keep a list of their names and telephone numbers.

- Keep your home safe and secure by installing deadbolt or slide-bolt locks on exterior doors and limiting access to potentially dangerous areas. Never lock the person with dementia in a home without supervision.

- Be aware that the person may not only wander by foot but also by car or by other modes of transportation.

*http://www.alz.org/Care/SafetyIssues/wandering.asp*

# "Oh my God! Where's Richard?"

I recently spent a week with my brother and his family. We see each other five or so times a year, and we frequently talk on the phone. He worries a lot about me.

Early in the visit, we spoke of my illness, but fortunately it did not seem to interfere with the rest of the visit.

One morning, I arose unusually early and ensconced myself in the bathroom at the far end of their house. As my brother and sister-in-law walked out of their bedroom, they noticed the door to my bedroom was open and I wasn't in there. They looked in the bathroom I had been using and I wasn't there. They each began to search the various rooms of the house, shouting, "Richard, Richard where are you?" I cracked open the door to the bathroom and replied, "I'm in here." Apparently, they didn't hear me. Suddenly, my brother rushed out of the house and started hollering, "Richard, Richard, where are you? Where are you? Where have you gone?" My sister-in-law rushed out of the back door of the house and began searching the backyard. Where was Richard? I put down the newspaper I was reading, leaned over, opened the door, and again said, "I'm in here!" Again, no one heard me.

I hurriedly finished my bathroom activities and came out and announced in a voice loud enough for both of them to hear: "I'm here, in the house." Both of them returned to the house and we all had a good laugh.

On a number of occasions, I've been separated from my wife in a mall and in large crowds. I never thought I was lost, but others assumed I had wandered off. We've all heard stories about people with Alzheimer's disease wandering into the neighbors' house and sleeping in their guest bed.

When I was first diagnosed with the disease, every time I got out of bed my wife

> When I was first diagnosed with the disease, every time I got out of bed my wife would inquire, "Where are you going?" I would tell her that I was going to wander naked around the neighborhood. We would both laugh, and she would fall back asleep.

would inquire, "Where are you going?" I would tell her that I was going to wander naked around the neighborhood. We would both laugh, and she would fall back asleep. The fear of wandering is real, both in me and in my caregivers. When I do wander off, it will be proof positive that I cannot take care of myself all of the time. It will be an incident that no one can or will ignore.

I was having a grand time with my brother and his family, just like the old days, and in walked Dr. Alzheimer with another glass of cold water to throw in my face. Although it ended up with us all laughing at ourselves and the situation, it revealed to me the underlying fear for me and my safety which is always in the hearts of my loved ones.

It is sad that I burden others with this fear. I so wish that it weren't so!

# This Little Light of Mine

What should I do with this the little light of mine—my experiences, insights, failures, and successes dealing with Alzheimer's disease? Should I hide my light under a bushel? Should I carry it all over the neighborhood, until somebody blows it out? Each of us has important insights into the Alzheimer's experience and because of the Alzheimer's experience. I believe the emotional pressure we all feel sometimes cracks through our own inhibitions, and we say and do things we would not otherwise say and do. In addition, we speak in ways we would not ordinarily speak. Sometimes, we are positively poetic! Moreover, we do not know or realize it.

There is a clarity, a universality of expression and meaning that speaks to everyone, a focus and elegance that for many of us, myself included, has managed to elude us most of our lives. All who are ingredients in the pressure cooker of Alzheimer's should write and share their thoughts and writings with others. E-mail them to family, whether or not they have asked for them. Send them as letters to the editor. Send a couple of them to your newspaper for inclusion in its "area" editions. Carry copies around with you, and if you strike up a conversation with someone and it seems appropriate, give them a copy of some of your writings.

> *All who are ingredients in the pressure cooker of Alzheimer's should write and share their thoughts and writings with others.*

I am not talking about writing down the details of the time you ran up and down the street naked or shouted "FREE POPCORN" in a crowded theater. I am talking about the way we speak and write about our experiences to each other, and frequently to ourselves, through journals and, now, blogs. Once the disease is conquered, and it *will* be at some future point in time, readers and writers will lose forever the sense of what it was like to live with *the* disease of probably the first 50 or so years of the 21st century. Pick up your pens, or sit down at your word processors. Think, feel, and write!

You are writing the poetry of Alzheimer's disease, only most of the time it does not rhyme. The definition of poetry is communication that evokes feeling, usually in verse form. For some reason, labeling a piece of writing as *poetry* often turns off most potential readers. I label the writings as poetry because the writing creates an emotional climate in which the description of even the most mundane of tasks becomes the communication of feeling.

If what you write is poetry or prose—well, that is of concern mostly to teachers of English. Miss Schetzel, my junior-year English teacher, might quibble with this, but years from now when Alzheimer's disease is a problem of the past, readers will look at the writings of the direct and indirect conscripts of Alzheimer's as powerful poetry. Love, fear, anger, and frustration are all expressed in their rawest, most human form.

All of us walking down Alzheimer Avenue should write about our experiences in order to feel freer; in fact, we should feel a sense of obligation to share our day with others. It is good for us, the writers, and good for the readers. There is clarity to life when life is at stake. Love and commitment ooze through the words of a frustrated daughter trying to get her Dad to stop driving. Self-doubt about whether he can really take care of his spouse of 30 years pungently seasons the description of a husband trying to figure out how to do the wash, when prior to this, *doing the wash* meant taking his socks out from under the bed and placing them in the clothes hamper.

Your writings will not end up in high school literature classes or in poetry books, but they have potentially profound value to all who are living today just like yesterday, and tomorrow just like today. We have the opportunity to offer others the opportunity to learn about themselves based on more than simply their own experience.

We do not feel more emotions, or even different emotions, than anyone else does. We may experience more of them at the same time than most people. We may experience them as all-consuming as an emotion can be to a human being. We are not special or unique, but we live within a special set of circumstances, which, thankfully, not all do. What we do and learn about ourselves, each other, and life is just as important to share as what William Shakespeare or Emily Dickinson shared. We may not be able to express ourselves in three unrhymed lines of five, seven, and five syllables (a haiku), but who, other than Miss Schetzel, is counting?

Hide it under a bushel? NO! I'm gonna let it shine. And you should, too!

*Give light, and the darkness will disappear of itself.*
—Desiderius Erasmus

# Am I To Be My Spouse's Son?

When I was a child, I thought as a child and I acted as a child. Now I am an adult. I think as an adult and I act as an adult. Unique to me, I think and act as an adult who has Alzheimer's disease. The fact that I have a disease affecting my memory and cognitive processes does not make me any less an adult or any more like a child. Why, then, do people choose to treat me like a child? Why do people slow down as they speak to me? Why do they shorten their sentences? Why do they keep repeating the same things over and over again?

Why do they act like an adult speaking to a child and expect me to act like a child speaking to an adult? Good question, and it is important for everyone who has and who communicates daily with someone who has Alzheimer's disease to try and answer. In fact, if one is to believe all this preaching about treating us with dignity and in ways that enhance our self-esteem, then caregivers' patterns of communication have a profound impact on those for whom they care.

One of the easiest ways for me to become angry is to perceive that someone is treating me like a child. "There, there, Richard, let me help you with that." "Don't touch that!" "Didn't I just tell you that?" "Now listen to me!" Unfortunately, from where I sit, there are no good models of behavior that we can observe as children and then apply as adults to interactions with older and younger adults who have some form of dementia. I remember how people treated my grandmother when she was 92 and I was seven years old. I see how people talk and behave around older people. I have visited Alzheimer's care facilities and watched staff and caregivers relate to the guests. Through my haze, the future looks bleak.

It is not so much *what* people say; it is how they say it. It is their body language. It is the look in their eyes as they lean slightly forward, place their hand on my elbow, look at me directly in the eyes in a way they would never look at another adult who did not have Alzheimer's, and slowly enunciate their words. They emphasize the end of each sentence. Sometimes they speak louder than usual, as if I am hearing impaired. Sometimes, there is a softness and lowered volume in their voice as if they do not want to wake me from my dreamland. When I say something, they respond with a smile and then continue their monologue as if I was watching their speech rather than participating in a conversation.

Honest, this happens to me once or twice a week, and I am only 62 years old and in the early stages of the disease. Imagine how often older people and people with more advanced stages of Alzheimer's must be on the receiving end of these kinds of well-intended but demeaning behaviors. What must they be thinking? How must they be feeling? It is little wonder that after a while, some people just seem to give up, become helpless, and "let" others treat them like babies.

The truth is that we do not know, nor will we ever know, their "musts" in terms of feeling and thinking. Right now, I can tell you my "musts," and you may not like what I have to say. I don't like being treated that way! What you sincerely and, from my perspective, thoughtlessly believe to be appropriate is demeaning, distracting, and does not help me feel good about you or myself.

> *I am not a child. Even if sometimes I act like one, check me out—I AM NOT A CHILD!*

I am not a child. Even if sometimes I act like one, check me out—I AM NOT A CHILD!

Now, having completed my childlike temper tantrum over how I don't want to be treated: How do I *want* to be treated? Dare I say, "I do not now know?" Is that a cop-out? Am I leaving it up to you to figure out for both of us how best to treat me in my later stages? Sort of! I believe we all need to develop a fresh approach to each other: one that we can discuss with each other as I change, and as you change; one that encourages me to be independent rather than dependent; one that helps me feel loved, not smothered; one that reminds me I am still an adult, not a child evolving into a helpless baby.

## THE ISSUES

I'm not you and never can be.
I'm not who you think I am.
I'm not who you want me to be.
I'm resisting some learned and deeply etched urge to become the me that you want.
Your current behavior isn't helping me be the me I want to be for as long as I want to, and for as long as I can.

It would be easier for both of us if I just "gave up" and you just
"gave in" and I became your younger and younger child and you
became my parent.
You are not me and never can be.

We are both unwilling conscripts and we both expend a lot of
energy being upset with each other: upset at being conscripted and
really upset because we were conscripted by this particular disease. The
enemy is not Dr. Alzheimer; he is dead, and the disease is something
neither of us can "behave" away. Wasting time wishing we would act
like each other or how the other would like us to act is truly a waste
of time.

## TALK WITH YOUR SPOUSE AND PARENTS NOW

Talking clearly and directly with your spouse and parents about their needs and your concerns can be an upsetting experience for all. Most aging people fear losing their independence and are anxious and sometimes fearful about what the future holds. An independent
and supportive spouse or parent may become pessimistic, demanding, and hard to deal with.
Without prior planning, you may find yourself handling an emergency situation without the
time and information needed to get the best help.

Learn of your spouse's and parent's wishes and their plans for the future. Many times,
adult children make assumptions about what parents want without asking them or listening
to their concerns. Treat your spouse or parent as a partner in decisions you must make together. A spouse or parent doesn't want to be treated like a child any more than you want to
play the role of parent.

*http://www.cope-inc.com/aging.html*

# Okay? Okay! *and* Okay.

People are always asking me: "Are you okay? Is (this or that) okay? Okay." Sometimes the *okay* seems to have a question mark after. Sometimes it seems to have an exclamation mark after it. And sometimes it seems to have a period after it.

It makes a big difference—punctuation, that is. The most difficult *okay* for me to deal with is the well-intended, "Okay!" When most people say it to me, they mean, "End of discussion." I am okay with it, now you be okay with it. Someone will say something to me and offer advice or answer a question and end the conversation with, "Okay!" To them it seems to mean I have answered the question, I have given you the right answer, so let's move on. "OKAY!" Just because I have Alzheimer's disease and ask you a question doesn't mean that whatever you say is okay with me. I just wanted to hear, but not necessarily follow, your advice.

I get a lot of these "Okay!"s. Well-meaning people are trying to make my life easier. When I pause to fish for a word, they catch it for me. When I am confused as to how to begin, they gently nudge me aside and start it for me, then turn to me and say, "Okay!" Seldom do they pause and ask me if what they did was okay with me. Most of the time, this works for me. It is no big deal if I cannot figure out how to put new string in the weed eater. I do not care if I can correctly recall my date of birth, Social Security number, and years at my present address. In fact, it is handy having human memory chips standing around apparently just waiting for the opportunity to fill in for my short-circuiting and gummed-up synapses. On the other hand, there are times when I want to figure things out for myself. There are times when, for reasons known only to my therapist and my subconscious, I am embarrassed because I cannot recall the name of my grandchildren or my daughter-in-law. I want to know that I know their names, and if it takes me a few extra seconds to find the names, please just stand around and wait with me until the correct answer comes out through my mouth. I realize this puts caregivers in the position of guessing. The best solution I can think of is to reduce the number of "OKAY!"s and turn them into "Okay?" Then, even if I wanted to figure it out, we can at least talk about our differing expectations.

The second type of *okay* ends with a question mark: "Okay?" I take that to mean that people are asking me if what they just did or said is okay with me. I like this one, most of the time. I am being asked to approve what has just happened. Did the other person get it right, from my perspective? Sometimes I still do not know if it is okay, but I assume they know or can recall more about the subject than I, so I nod my head approvingly. Sometimes I didn't want them to solve the problem for me, I just wanted to hear their thinking. I didn't need the complete answer from their perspective, just some additional information. The question mark sometimes means *yes* or *no*, when all I want to convey is *okay*.

Once in a great while, the *okay* ends with a period. I wish I heard more of these. I wish I were more open to asking for help. I wish my caregivers were more open to first asking me if I wanted help, instead of assuming that every time I paused or seemed confused it was their obligation to step in and help me. Okay! Now, caregivers, you read my mind and know if I want an *Okay!* an *Okay?* an *Okay.* or just silence, and let me figure it out for myself.

When an *okay* comes with a period, I take that as meaning *I finished what I wanted to say, I finished what I wanted to do, and to me it is okay. Now the ball is in your court to respond to my* okay. *You can assume it is okay and not say anything, and we can move on. You can confirm the* okay *with an* okay *of your own. On the other hand, you can proclaim that it is not okay, and tell me your reasons for rejecting my* okay.

For most readers, this may appear to be much ado about nothing. For people with Alzheimer's, *okay* is a very powerful word. We know that physiologically we are not okay. Psychologically, we struggle with our personal okayness. You are okay because you don't have Alzheimer's disease. I am not okay because I do. Emotionally, I am frequently looking for affirmation and support from others to reassure me that what I do and say is okay. I do not want to be told things are okay just because you said it was okay. I do not want to be embarrassed by being asked if something is okay when obviously I did not understand it in the first place—unless I am in a particularly well-balanced moment of my life and okay with it.

> *You are okay because you don't have Alzheimer's disease. I am not okay because I do.*

Okay! Get it? I think it best if we all stop saying "Okay" to each other and say what we really mean.

# Have You Ever Participated
## in One of These Conversations?

I don't believe he has lung cancer. I cough just like he does!
I don't believe my mom has Alzheimer's. I forget my keys, too, and
sometimes I get confused.

He doesn't have a genetic disorder. He has a blood disease. I know
one when I see it.
He doesn't have Alzheimer's disease. He has a mental problem, if
you know what I mean.

He can't have diabetes! He is too young.
He can't have Alzheimer's disease! He is too young.

Why should I get a power of attorney now? Huntington's disease
will take years to end her life.
Why should I get a power of attorney now? Alzheimer's disease isn't
affecting her mind!

I saw her in the mall! She didn't look like she had breast cancer.
I saw her in the mall. She didn't look like she had Alzheimer's disease.

I just spoke with her on the phone. She didn't sound like she had
leukemia.
I just spoke with her on the phone. She didn't sound like she had
Alzheimer's disease.

You don't look like you had your spleen removed to me.
You don't look confused, disoriented, and/or lost to me.

You know, it's hard for me to tell the difference between a heart attack and indigestion.
You know, it's hard for me to tell the difference between Alzheimer's disease and just plain growing old.

Isn't everyone going to get malaria sometime in their life? What's
the big deal?
Isn't everyone going to get Alzheimer's disease? What's the big
deal?

You look great: haven't changed since I saw you last month. I guess all that stuff about hepatitis C was a bunch of crap.

You look great: haven't changed since I saw you last month. I guess your Alzheimer's disease hasn't progressed.

I have an Aunt who had what I believe was a common cold. Strangest thing, she coughed, sneezed, looked run down, had a rash, lacked coordination, and coughed up blood (these are signs of a form of atypical pneumonia).

I have an Aunt who has what I believe is Alzheimer's disease. Strangest thing—she thinks she is a teapot.

I'll be honest with you. I don't think our brother has colon cancer. I think he has a reoccurring case of flatulence, and this Doctor is trying to make a buck off us.

I'll be honest with you. I don't think our brother has Alzheimer's disease. I think he is just growing old before his time, and this Doctor is trying to make a buck off us.

I thought only young people had to watch what they ate. Hell, I'm too old to worry about cholesterol. I'm just a little tired from eating so much at the fish fry.

I thought only old people got Alzheimer's disease. Hell, she's 40 years old. Why should we even be talking about this? She is just plain off her rocker.

# Is It Okay To Say You Have a "Touch" of Alzheimer's?

While shopping in a large department store, I approached the checkout counter. The associate behind the counter was obviously confused as to how to ring up a credit for returned merchandise, and then take that credit and apply it to the cost of merchandise that the customer wanted to purchase using her credit card. He looked around, saw me waiting impatiently for him to figure it out, and said, "Pardon me; I must have a touch of Alzheimer's today." No one waiting in line laughed out loud. A few smiled, and several nodded approvingly as if to say, "It has happened to me, too."

If I accidentally dropped a cup of coffee on your brand-new white carpet, would it be appropriate for me to say, "Excuse me, I think I have a touch of Huntington's disease today"? If, while playing tennis with you, I requested a short break between the games because I was feeling a little shaky and not in control of some of my muscles, would you smile if I said, "I feel just like I have a touch of Parkinson's disease"? If I fell down and hit my head on the sidewalk, would people smile when I said, touching the lump on the back of my head, "Why, I feel like I have a tumor from a fast-growing form of brain cancer"?

Is it appropriate to use the name of the disease to describe a temporary and vaguely similar set of symptoms in a healthy person? Especially a disease that shortens people's lives, strips them of all dignity as they near the moment of death, and absorbs their personality and identity and replaces it with a blank stare for the last year or so of their lives? When I show up for dinner with my shirt incorrectly buttoned, my family and I share a laugh as I re-button the shirt. Moreover, if I re-buttoned it wrong a second time, we laugh even louder. How would I feel if I walked into a room full of strangers with my shirt incorrectly buttoned and they all started to laugh at me? How do I feel when, in casual conversation, other people profess to have a touch of Alzheimer's disease? Honestly, it makes me mad—or, as my therapist would encourage me to characterize it, "I make myself mad when other people—who do not appreciate the enormity of the disease and are not intimately involved with it—use Alzheimer's as a source of humor." Who is right and who is wrong? Who is not sensitive enough, and who is too sensitive?

The answer is probably both of us. I can't expect other people to appreciate this disease in the way that I do. They can't expect me to appreciate what they really mean when they say, "I have a touch of Alzheimer's." It is pretty much a universal theme of humor to laugh at people who are inebriated. As someone who is drunk slurs their speech, staggers down the street, and becomes confused as to where he or she lives, most of us chuckle. I wonder if every member of Alcoholics Anonymous is chuckling right along with us. Adults who have recently experienced the death of a loved one watch and, I suspect, feel uncomfortable, sad, and sometimes angry as a "funny" scene in a funeral home unfolds on a TV sitcom.

There is a saying: "Those who laugh, last." I am all for laughing. I think it is good for the soul, the spirit, the brain, and the heart. If we can't laugh at ourselves, will we ever have a right to laugh *with* others? Right now, about the only time I can laugh at myself is when I am with family. Even then, I must admit, I am a little uneasy, but I do see humor in my inability to correctly button my shirt. I am no authority on what is funny, why it is funny, and when it is okay and not okay to laugh. I am simply sensitized about something because I am experiencing it firsthand.

Perhaps we should exclude diseases as humorous or offhanded explanations for our behaviors. How does someone who has wrestled with serious manic depression for 20 years feel when someone says off-handedly, "I just feel manic today." The difference between laughing with someone and at someone is a personal perception. In the interests of other people whose sensitivity we do not know or appreciate, perhaps it would be best not to smile and certainly never to laugh aloud when it is possible that they are exhibiting the manifestation of a disease in their behavior. I am being polite and wordy with this because I can appreciate that it is hard for others to feel as I do. I wish others would grant me the same broad right. In addition, we would all protect each other's sensitivities and feelings.

> *I am no authority on what is funny, why it is funny, and when it is okay and not okay to laugh. I am simply sensitized about something because I am experiencing it firsthand.*

No more "A guy walks into a bar . . ." or "I feel like I have a touch of Alzheimer's." There is a lot in this world we can all laugh at that does not approach the line of sarcasm and ridicule, regardless of our life circumstances. There are many other ways to rationalize away and dismiss our foibles without attributing them to diseases that people within hearing distance may be dealing with.

It's just too risky to say, and for many, myself included, it's just not funny!

---

For today I'd like to suggest that you use your power of humor to laugh at yourself. Laughter is one of the best forms of natural meditation. It improves the immune system, lowers blood pressure and diminishes the effects of stress. One major problem with the world is that we all take ourselves miles too seriously. We tend to think that life itself is a very grim and sober affair. We do not realize that the Creator is full of joy and sees the universe as a fun place. Just look at all the different animals in the world or the different people to notice that the Creator has a great sense of humor.

It is important that our laughter be loving and compassionate. Thus we would laugh with people rather than at them. The same attitude holds when we laugh at ourselves. I use the word "at" since that is the accepted usage but the attitude is to joyfully celebrate our own situation.

*http://www.lifefocuscenter.com/boostyourselfesteem703.htm*

# *Here! Take This!*

Most individuals, myself included, living with a diagnosis of Alzheimer's disease soon reach the point where they consume a handful of pills for breakfast and a handful and a half for dinner, and sometimes a couple of pills on an empty stomach as a late-night dessert. Caregivers order, pay for, inventory, sort, and pass out hundreds of them over the course of a month, and perhaps thousands of them over the course of a year. It becomes a big-time logistics operation: sorting Grandpa's pills into the little plastic boxes, each with three compartments. It must be frustrating to caregivers— at least once a week, I forget to take some pills, and I don't remember I forgot until someone sees the half-full box.

Over time, caregivers adjust to their responsibilities, but sometimes the consumers of these pills do not.

"I don't need any pills."

"I don't like to take them."

"*You* take them if they are so good for me."

Sometimes a handful of pills is met with sealed lips and a hard, cold stare.

Caregivers respond with

"Please?"

"These are for your own good."

"Here."

"The doctor said to take these, NOW!"

"Here!"

"Do you want to feel better?"

"Here! Now take these! Now! I haven't got any more time to waste messing around with you and your pills!"

"I sort 'em, now you swallow 'em!"

Caregivers try reason, pleading, distracting, joking, demanding, and whatever button worked the last time, they push it again. A caregiver, who is a close friend of mine, told me he once found himself on his knees in front of his 85-year-old mom with a handful of pills, raised as if they were the Holy Eucharist, saying: "Take and eat. These are your pills, I have purchased for thee" (or words to that effect).

The dictionary offers several definitions of "pill." Sometimes two definitions seem to be true at the same time.

> pill
> 1a : medicine in a small rounded mass to be swallowed whole
> 4 : a disagreeable or tiresome person

Personally, I have no objection to taking my pills. Why is it, then, when somebody reminds me I haven't taken my pills this morning or evening I say, "Okay," and then they remind me again 30 minutes later. Why do I sometimes forget to take my pills? And, while we're on the subject, what is it with caregivers that makes the taking of pills a matter of life or death? Personally, I think it has nothing to do with pills. I know for some of us they are painful to swallow, but for all they

> *The longer I live with Alzheimer's disease, the less important the pills become to me.*

are a painful sign that we must and do swallow them twice a day. I suspect that not taking my meds is my way of saying "NO" to the disease. It is my way of remaining in control of me. I'll determine what, when, and where I put something in my mouth. It is my way of saying, "That's enough for now. Enough is enough." For many who are farther down the line, it is a way of saying, "I have already given up. Can't you understand that these pills are helping you, not me! I don't want to go on any longer and, to the extent these pills are making that happen, I want to put a stop to it."

The longer I live with Alzheimer's disease, the less important the pills become to me. The farther along I am into the disease, the more important the pills become to my caregivers. I want them to understand that I don't want to swallow a bitter pill twice a day—nor do I want to be the bitter pill my caregivers must swallow every day.

So how many pills are consumed by us over the course of one year? Some guy paid Google $50 to answer this question:

*How many tablets/pills are produced annually in the US?*

*This would include pharma based drugs (generic and branded), OTC (over-the-counter drugs) and supplements/vitamins (nutraceuticals).*

*Number of pills would be great—value of the pills also would be nice.*

*Also, bonus information would include what percent are specifially colored/branded with a color or other effect.*

Google couldn't find out the answer but charged him $50 just for looking. One plant in Thailand has the capacity for producing 1 billion pills a year, so you can start there with your own estimates.

# *What Is It Like Not To Have Alzheimer's Disease?*

I had a bittersweet experience this morning. For almost five hours, everyone in the world responded to me as if I did not have Alzheimer's disease. It felt wonderful! People looked directly at me and looked directly into my eyes when they spoke to me. People instigated casual conversation with me. People treated me like I was independent, competent, knowledgeable, and important. People depended on me. People listened to me. People responded to me as if I were a husband, a full family member, and a responsible adult.

For the past three weeks my wife, my best friend, my lover, my chief caregiver has been living with the pain of a bulging disk in her back. Finally, after three weeks of pain, five prescriptions, and swallowing 10 pounds of pills, each and all of which had no effect on her pain, she allowed herself to be scheduled for a procedure which injected medication directly into the site of her pain (between L4 and L5).

My daughter-in-law drove us to the outpatient surgical center. We were pre-registered, so there was no paperwork to complete. As we walked back to the O.R. patient preparation area, nurses and technicians started to ask me questions. "How long did she have the pain? Was it a burning sensation? Did the pain run down along one of her legs? Was she allergic to any drugs?" She could have answered any of these questions herself, but since she winced in pain with every step she took, people addressed their questions to me. I don't know what was more amazing to me, knowing the answers or being asked the questions.

I helped her out of her clothes and into her gown. As we waited in this little room for the doctor to arrive, more people came in and asked me questions! Oh, it felt so good to help my wife, and for my word to be taken as the truth. Everyone seemed to rely on my answers. There were no knowing glances to other people in the room, seeking confirmation of my answers. I was back in the game of life again!

The doctor walked in and started to speak to my wife, and after her fourth or fifth wince of pain brought on by her back spasms, he turned to me. What did we know about her condition, and what were our expectations of this procedure? It had been a long time since someone had inquired of *me* what my wife and I knew about something. People had long ago ceased to ask me what Linda and I felt about something as a couple. Inquiries are now directed almost exclusively to Linda. What did *she* know? How did *she* feel? *What's going on with Richard?*

About halfway into my response to the doctor's question, "What do you know about her condition?" the doctor interrupted me and asked me a question. I actually knew more, thanks to the Internet and Mr. Google, than he did, albeit about a minor point dealing with her condition. I vaguely recall a time when lots of people were coming to me and asking for information and my opinion concerning things other than myself or my disease. It felt wonderful to be back there again—a credible player in the game.

> *I vaguely recall a time when lots of people were coming to me and asking for information and my opinion concerning things other than myself or my disease. It felt wonderful to be back there again.*

As they were preparing to take Linda to the O.R., the doctor turned to me and asked me a question about myself. Someone outside of my family and friends was interested in me; not my condition, not the disease, not what it felt like to have Alzheimer's disease. He asked me a question about me! Was I from Chicago? He was from Chicago! He lived on the North Side near Wrigley Field, just like me. At last a conversation about nothing, and I was half of the conversation!

I didn't fully appreciate this entire experience until we returned home, where everybody knows both my name and my disease. People treated me as if I overslept and didn't go to the surgical center.

What happened? How did it go? My daughter-in-law became the preferred source of information. People called and talked to her. People visited and looked her in her eyes. People took her at her word.

It was a wonderful morning I shall not soon forget—I hope!

# There Is Something (More) Wrong with Dad

⋊⋈⋊⊹⋈⋊⊹⋈⋊⊹⋈⋊

Almost four years ago I started strolling down the road, arm and arm with Dr. Alzheimer. My daughter signaled the start when, after a visit with us, she whispered in my wife's ear as we drove to the airport, "There is something wrong with Dad." Four years later and there is now hesitancy in my walk. I'm not as sure of my steps as I was at the start. I know how to act like I did at the start, but sometimes I slip up and am unaware of the slip. I can't seem to close the increasingly widening gap between my caregivers and me. We don't talk as openly or as much about what is going on with me. They talk more about me without me. They worry more about me. They watch what I do more. They comment more often on my mistakes: "You left the stove on." "You are wearing your shirt inside out. It is buttoned wrong." "Did you call this person, like I asked you to?" Perhaps they are still responding to the same percentage of mistakes, but it is just that I am making more of them. I'm not sure.

Sometimes, in the heat of the moment I blurt out something that later I wish I had not blurted. Sometimes, in the heat of the moment a truth is revealed to me that would not otherwise have so clearly revealed itself had I not been in the midst of a heated moment. You decide. I'm not sure.

I love working in my garden. I love the process of preparing the soil, planting seeds, nurturing plants, watching them grow, harvesting them, and either watching them die, in the case of flowers, or eating them, in the case of vegetables. This year's garden is not as successful as last year's garden. Nor was last year's garden as successful as the year before. While I still love working in the garden, I'm less organized, less focused, less attentive, less careful, less concerned, and you get it—each year, I'm less and less competent as a master gardener. While some of my family enjoy my flowers, and some of my family enjoy eating my vegetables, no one in my family enjoys working with me in the garden. I imagined Grandpa sitting there on his stool passing on his gardening knowledge to his grandchildren and watching them scurry about the flower-filled garden. It was just in my imagination. There are bugs in the garden—vicious and aggressive bugs. There is a persistent rumor that there is a snake in the garden, as yet unconfirmed by an actual sighting. There are plants with stickers in the garden. Unfortunately, these rumors and fears are enough to keep my grandchildren hiding behind their parents as they stand and watch me and my garden.

This year, I announced that I was not going to garden any more. I would transplant my roses and perennials along the side of the fence, cut up the rails that created my elevated garden, and gently slope the garden soil toward our property line.

Upon making this announcement to my family, everyone (except me) attended a meeting whose sole agenda item seemed to be how to rationalize my decision to discontinue my garden as not being their fault. Each attendee then found me alone for a moment and told me that it was not his or her fault that no one supported my garden, and how they wished they could have, but they had some good excuse not to.

There is still something wrong with Dad. He is too sensitive; and besides, we never criticized. He is too defensive; and besides, we never accused him of anything. He changes his mind, and we don't. He gets his feelings hurt too easily, and we never intended that to happen. He doesn't understand, and we all do. Sometimes he's impossible to please, and we can't understand because we have never experienced that. There is something wrong with Dad. He loves his garden, but we don't have time to help him. And besides, we don't like to work in the garden. He knows that. He makes too many demands on us. We try to please him, but we can't please him all the time. And every time we fail to meet his expectations, which, by the way, are not always clear, he takes it personally. Just because something is important to him, he expects us to drop everything and

> *There is still something wrong with dad. He is too sensitive; and besides, we never criticized.*

make it equally important to us. Just because he had to wait a while for us to answer one of his requests, he expects us to appreciate even more the fact that we are meeting his request. Just because he can't drive, we should drive him whenever and wherever he wants. Just because he can't garden as well as he did in the past, we should act as his assistant gardener. Just because he has Alzheimer's disease and we don't, etc. . . ."

Is something more wrong with Dad? Is it the same problem, only more of it? You decide. I'm not sure. And more frightening to me is the fact I can't be sure if I am unsure or not!

P.S. Now, "Where was the moment of clarity?" you may still be asking yourself. It came after I wrote this! Increasingly, my family and I are lapsing into a them versus me, or a me versus them, mentality. One side is right and I am wrong, or I am right and they are clearly wrong. Questions of right and wrong may be clear to the President of the United States, but to folks with Alzheimer's disease it is the wrong frame, the wrong question, the wrong time, and the wrong way to resolve common problems.

It isn't a compromise where I give up something and they give up something. It isn't giving in where I get what I want and they don't get what they want. We all want the same thing! The only problem is that we sometimes want a thing to the exclusion of what the other person wants. We all want to make the best of this terrible situation. We all want what is best for each other and ourselves. We all want to be as happy as circumstances (and we) will allow ourselves to be. We don't necessarily want to be right or wrong. We just act that way! We shouldn't. There is no one best way to solve a problem; it is best when everyone agrees it is best, not because it just is.

Everyone gives lip service to more communication, more open communication, more two-way communication. Unless we all still speak from our hearts, from the love and respect we have for each other, all these communication strategies are a way to avoid fundamental issues. Do we love each other? Are we willing to sacrifice our wants for the wants of someone we profess to love? Are we in this together for the long haul, or the short fix? Increasingly, there is something wrong with all of us! Although we can all respond to these questions in a rational and affirmative manner, why undermine our shared foundation by stepping away from our love and joining the debate team?

> *Everyone gives lip service to more communication, more open communication, more two-way communication.*

# Time to Clean Up Your Act

Although yet to be a major issue in my life, bathing, personal hygiene, hair washing, and general cleanliness are issues I know are on the minds and in the hearts and noses of many, many caregivers. A quick-and-dirty content analysis of over 1,000 postings in three different Internet chat rooms composed primarily of caregivers of individuals with Alzheimer's revealed that personal hygiene was a close second to eating as the most frequently mentioned issue.

It has been my experience that people who have jobs develop routines that revolve around their jobs. People who don't have jobs have nothing around which they can build a routine. If I awake at 10:30 A.M., or noon, or 7 P.M., I am still faced with the same set of choices. What am I going to do next? In my working days, I knew what I had to do next: take the dog out to pee, take a shower, shave, brush my teeth, dress, etc.

In my current world, my routine grows only out of the need for my dog to relieve herself. Usually, I take her outside in the morning. Sometimes, I forget and she reminds me. If she doesn't want to "go," we both sleep in and she skips peeing and I skip my shower. No big deal.

Here I go again, offering more information than you need or, dare I say, want to know, and I have yet to get to my point.

Family members go to great lengths not to have to say to a senior family member, "You smell." It is not really about the odor, or so they say. They tell each other they are concerned that my new-found odor has been caused by unclean habits. Perhaps my body is teeming with flesh-eating bacteria, or the Ebola virus, or even worse, body odor-causing germs.

> *Family members go to great lengths not to have to say to a senior family member, "You smell."*

In my opinion, family members spend a lot of unnecessary time worrying about how bad Dad or Mom smells. Family members scheme amongst themselves, looking for ways to get around having to confront someone living with a disease of dementia over the issue of cleanliness. Leaving extra deodorant sticks in the bathroom, asking if they've run out of soap, offering to help them with a shower or bath, announcing that "something smells in here" and then pretending they don't know what it is—these are none-too-subtle ways of avoiding having to say, "Why can't you smell/be like me?"

I believe that the "problem" of cleanliness is greatly exaggerated by caregivers. I believe this is an example of a misplaced concern. I believe this is an example of a stalking horse (B.O.) substituting for some real and more important issues. Of all the concerns churning between family members and within each of the family members, personal choices concerning personal hygiene are relatively low on my priority list, especially when many other issues higher on the list are ignored.

Now, I'm not advocating that I be encouraged to wear vomit-crusted shirts and to walk on a feces-covered rug. I'm just talking about my body odor, the fact that I don't shave every day like I did when I was younger and employed, my lack of concern with how my hair looks to other people, if my clothes match, if I do or do not wear my bottom dental plate and if I brush it more than once at Christmas: These should all be of little concern to you, and of minor concern to me. Why, then, is there so much focus on how I smell and why I smell? If I don't sense or believe I smell or, in your words, "smell awful," and I spend 24 of every 24 hours a day home with myself, why should your issue rise to the level of a family crisis? I don't smell like you, I don't want to smell like you, and if truth be known, I never wanted to smell like you! You wear far too much perfume. People can smell you 5 minutes before you walk into a room and 30 minutes after you have left. You wear too much after-shave lotion, and it makes my eyes water when you lean over to hug me. No one should walk around smelling like a musk ox or a spring rain shower.

*Treat us as someone you love as we are, not who you wish we were or who you want and think we should be.*

You know, if we would only be more open, more honest, and more fact-based in all our conversations concerning my illness, it would be much easier for all of us to deal with this issue. If nothing is truly wrong with me, if I am just a little forgetful, if it's none of your business, why is everyone so constipated because I stopped washing and combing my hair?

Because there is so little that can be done to attack the disease itself, a lot of misplaced energy goes into attacking the consequences of the disease. We should wash clean our list of concerns and first deal with the facts of my disease. We don't need to label it; just help me and, by the way, you understand that I have it, I'm not alone, and people still love me.

Caregivers stress themselves as much or more than do the people for whom they care. We can't be who you want or need us to be. Don't get upset with us or yourself when we aren't. Treat us as someone you love *as we are*, not who you wish we were or who you want and think we should be. We don't intend to make you mad just being ourselves; we don't go out of our way to make you mad. You push us to be as you are and we push back. You push us to be as we were and we don't understand.

Remember, you are the one with the upsetting problem. I like the way I smell, I don't care how I smell, and/or I never thought about it. I have other things I deem more important on my mind, and so should you.

## TRAVELING

Do not negotiate an outing with a person with dementia. Instead of asking, "Are you ready to go out?" limit what he or she must remember by announcing "Here's your coat" and "We're getting into the car now."

Reassure the person. New and different surroundings can be anxiety producing and disorienting for someone with dementia.

Plan your route as carefully as you can, know about parking, elevators, stairs, and so forth. Leave plenty of time so you will not need to rush.

If taking a vacation or weekend away with someone with dementia, consider bringing along another adult to help out. Bring something to help keep the confused person occupied if you must wait somewhere. Try a package of snacks, cards, or a picture book.

*http://www.zarcrom.com/users/alzheimers/c-07.html*

# "Don't Worry About Anything. We'll Take Care of It."

*Just because you're paranoid, it doesn't mean
they're not out to get you.*
—Unknown

I am presently in the midst of my second circuit visiting the various members of my family in their own homes. This time, I am staying longer than my previous visit. Everyone tells me this "vacation is for my own good—to give me a break" from the caregivers with whom I interact on a daily basis in and around my own home.

"Oh," say I.

I was told that I was the one who suggested this, and everyone is cooperating because, after all, "this would give everyone a break from each other."

Oh?

It is true that I suggested it was time for me to travel. I had been told over and over what a strain my behaviors and attitudes were having on my caregivers. I had been told I needed to change my ways in order for them to feel less stressed. I was told they couldn't change much or any more than they already had, and I was being unrealistic, demanding, and selfish when I kept expecting and asking for others to adjust to me and my disease. They had already adjusted, and to ask for more, to expect more, to be disappointed when it didn't happen (the changes I was demanding/asking) created stress of unimaginable proportions. I had become my own worst problem and the primary cause of many other people's stress.

Given this environment and having been labeled as the chief cause of stress in a family that was already stressed out, is it any wonder I suggested that perhaps this would be a good time for me to pack my bags and get out of town. Was this suggestion free from coercion? No!

"Oh!"

"And, by the way, this will give you a needed rest from us as much as it will give us a needed rest from you," say my caregivers. Sort of like a reciprocal respite from each other and for each other.

Oh?

"And don't worry about bringing any money; we will pay all your expenses. We will feed you. We will entertain you. We want to!" say they.

"Well, what about my desire to give you some money for food? I would like to take you out to eat once in a while. What if I need a hair-cut? What if I want to buy a present or two to take back to my grand-children?" ask I.

"Don't worry, we will take complete care of you!" say they.

"Well, what if I don't *want* my family to take 'complete care' of me just yet? What if I want to maintain some feeling of independence?" ask I.

"Why, we want you to feel loved and well taken care of. It would be an honor for us to give back to you, to include you in our family activities," say they.

"Thank you. And what about my need and desire to maintain some of my own independence and feel and act like I am an almost completely functioning adult? What about some sort of compromise wherein we could both feel and respect each other's and our own needs and wants?" ask I.

"Don't worry, we always have your best interests in mind, and we can and will take care of everything," say they.

> And what about my need and desire to maintain some of my own independence and feel and act like I am an almost completely functioning adult?

"Will you please work with me to find ways to enable me to do more, rather than disable me to do less?" plead I.

"Don't worry, we have your best interests at heart. You haven't done well in the past at handling money. You don't need to. We will take care of everything."

"Oh."

I know and feel that each and every member of my family loves me, respects me, and wants me to be happy. I know in their hearts they strongly believe they are doing what is best for me. It is clear to me: They either don't understand what I am saying or asking for, or they believe they know what is best for me despite my protestations, or they are so overwhelmed by their own fears, stress, diversions, or lives that they cannot or will not consider any concerns other than their own. Or, perhaps it is a combination of these. Or, perhaps it is some factor to which I am blind.

I can't get inside their heads like they can't get inside mine. We all remain connected through our hearts, but this connection is increasingly strained by our lack of connection through our brains.

What to do? Who will do it? When will they do it so it will benefit all, especially me?

General wording: "Do unto others as you would have them do unto you."

Christianity: "Therefore all things whatsoever ye would that men should do to you, do ye even so to them." (Matthew 7:12)

Judaism: "Thou shalt love thy neighbor as thyself." (Leviticus 19:18)

Islam: "No one of you is a believer until he loves for his brother what he loves for himself."

Confucianism: "What you do not want done to yourself, do not do to others." (Analects 15:23)

Buddhism: "Hurt not others with that which pains yourself." (Udanavarga 5:18)

Hinduism: "Good people proceed while considering that what is best for others is best for themselves." (Hitopadesa)

Humanism: "Every person has dignity and worth, and, therefore, should command the respect of every other person." (This is in contrast to medieval scholars who taught that life on Earth was to be despised and that humans were sinful creatures who should be devoting their lives to getting into heaven.)

Communist motto: "From each according to his ability, to each according to his needs."

Indian saying: "Don't judge others until you have walked in their moccasins."

# Should We Do unto Others
# What We Perceive They Have
# Already Done unto Us?

Everyone needs a philosophy of life. Mental health is
based on the tension between what you are and
what you think you should become. You should
be striving for worthy goals. Emotional
problems arise from being purposeless.

—Viktor Frankl (1970)

O n-line chat support groups all over the world wrestle with postings that include unfavorable remarks (some would characterize them as attacks) about other participants' politics and
religion. The "moderators" of these rooms (those who are actually
running the rooms) sometimes electronically ban people from return-
ing to that Internet site.

One of the rooms for which I am one of four moderators recently
confronted this issue when one of the participants made several dis-
paraging remarks about the intellectual capacity of the President of
the United States. One of the moderators (not yours truly) posted a
public reprimand of the criticizer. This was my response to my fellow
chat-room posters on the subject of tolerance.

There are no emotional "depends" we can all wear so when the
stress of having Alzheimer's, or of taking care of someone with this
disease, causes us to have a bad moment or a bad day. We are always
responsible for our own behaviors, even when we want to take them
back. We should say, "I'm sorry; it was not you, it was me. I don't
know where that came from." If we criticize another person, if we call
them names, speak ill of their intelligence, etc., is it my place to stand
up and say, "Stop. You are or might be offending others with your
judgments." If we use language that some find offensive, refer to religious beliefs of others without the same deference that believers at-

tribute to the words, is this grounds to dismiss the offender from the group? "No!" say I.

Keep your mind and your eye on why you are here. Do and say unto others as you would have them say and do unto you. And, if they don't, *don't* kick them out! Because we have been volunteered for the Alzheimer's experience is not a justification to abandon our lifelong quest to live a well-examined life. Even if it was not Adam and Eve's fault, we are all not perfect! How much energy we invest in our quest for perfection depends in large degree, I believe, on how much stress is in our life. Right now, we cannot afford to sit in a hole in the ground in India and ponder our perfection or lack thereof. We are on the front lines of human emotional turmoil! We are at war with disease! Moreover, we know we are going to lose! This is a pretty good explanation of why we do what we do, but it is not an excuse to abandon lifelong relationships, friendships, our quest to understand ourselves, and whatever commitment we have made to whomever (ourselves included) to give the best of ourselves and expect nothing (or, at least, no more than a little) in return.

I am willing to cut some slack to those, myself included, in the Alzheimer's pressure cooker. It isn't fair, it isn't right, and I don't like it. Sometimes I can't handle it by myself, and I say things which, at the time, seemed like the right thing to say. I don't intend to cause harm with my words, but sometimes I am convinced, at least for the moment, that something has to be said. Sometimes I don't even go through all these mental gyrations, I just blurt out something that in other circumstances I'd know would be hurtful, but now I feel so hurt I override the "Do unto others" circuit with a large charge of ME!

When I cannot figure something out, my first reaction is to proclaim, "Give me a break. I am the one with Alzheimer's." I have actually

> *I am really not sure that if I did* not *have Alzheimer's, I still wouldn't have reacted the same way, but that is an issue for my therapist, pastor, and God to deal with.*

said this, I am not proud to report. Sometimes that is even my second, third, and fourth reactions. Usually, I can figure out what happened—eventually. Sometimes, dare I say, I can't or *won't*, and I just move on and leave unaddressed hurt feelings in others. I am really not sure that if I did *not* have Alzheimer's, I still wouldn't have reacted the same way, but that is an issue for my therapist, pastor, and God to deal with. Right now, I know I must try harder during those periods when I am "all here." I am trying, but sometimes I fail.

If a political opinion of mine or a religious belief of mine leaks into an on-line posting . . . so be it. We are still adults, and our collective goal should be to act like adults even if we believe someone else is not.

Please, everyone, chill out for a day before you start climbing in holes, leaving, or getting upset. We are all doing our best at any moment of the day, and sometimes our best doesn't work for others. As these are the times that try our souls, even our best is sometimes not good enough for us, let alone others. We don't have to discuss anything, but we should be able to say anything. Stop reading it, if you feel yourself getting upset. This isn't about you, it is about the person posting it, and the poster doesn't even really know you except for the few words you have written and posted here.

And, when these words did not ring reasonable and true, I tried:

Let's not let this devil stand up. Walk away from it, but stay here. Who among us thought everyone was going to like us and what we believed for the rest of our lives? We are all prone to project our own disappointments with the world, God, Dr. Alzheimer, or George Bush on to someone who at least we think we know. Now is *not* the time for us to look around for someone, something, some words to get mad at and feel offended by. Our own reality is enough to deal with, thank you. If others stray into bad habits, they only do so as a means of diverting their own pain and stress away from them and toward others.

If we didn't bring up God from time to time, we would stifle who we are, what we are thinking about, and how we feel. He, She, or It is part of most of our Alzheimer's stew. If we didn't mention something other than our own plight from time to time, we would implode; so, political comments will come and go.

We aren't angels! This isn't heaven! We shouldn't expect everyone else to be as close to being an angel as we are. As we *think* we are. As we want *others* to think we are. As we want others to be. As we know we are or aren't.

# When Most All Has
# Been Said, Little Has Been Done

*Why can't you please just be like me?*
*Really now, is that asking too much?*

After reading over 60,000+ words of mine, do you know what I really want and need? I will tell you. All I want, all I need, all I ask for is that others, especially my caregivers, be more like me. Not to act like me, but to understand me as I understand myself. I just want others to anticipate my needs and wants. I just want others to try every day to figure me out, to understand me. I just want others to love me as I love them.

Still confused, idealistic, unrealistic, and contradictory, aren't I?

I know I have a difficult mind to read. But, understand that is not my intent nor my fault. I didn't ask for this disease. I'm trying my best—are you? Or, are you so wrapped up in your own life and cares that you are unwilling to put your own needs on hold in order to first figure out and meet my needs? Do you so want me to be my former self that you look only for those signs, and miss who I am now?

Now, wanting everyone to be like me is not unique to having Alzheimer's disease. I said I wanted to marry someone who was, in most ways, different from me. Who would want to marry themselves? How boring! I found the woman of my dreams, and since our first disagreement (which occurred five minutes after we met, on our first date: "Where should we eat?"), I have spent large portions of the rest of my life trying to change her to be more like me. I have long since abandoned any hope of her ever being just like me. But, of course, that hasn't stopped me from trying!

When I first heard of my diagnosis, I remember thinking to myself, "How fortunate am I to have raised independent, free-thinking children and to have married a strong-willed, independent woman. They will make the hard decisions for me, the right decisions. They will take care of me!" Yes, they are taking care of me, but sometimes not in ways I want!

218

Sometimes their jobs, their own families, school, TV(!), or other obligations get in the way of doing what I thought we had all agreed they would do. Sometimes they do what we agreed they would do, but they do it wrong. They don't do it my way! Sometimes they just refuse to do what I think is right! Sometimes they forget, but I remember! Sometimes they agree, sort of, but I know they don't mean it in the same way I do. Perhaps worst of all, sometimes they put off even discussing it until some murky point in the distant future: "We will talk about it later." "We'll see." (That last one was one of my favorites as a parent, and I fear they have learned it from ME!).

So, what I have learned from thinking, writing, rethinking, rewriting, and rewriting and again reading 60,000 of my own well-chosen words?

I am as scared of the future as are my caregivers. We are afraid for different reasons, so it is very difficult for us to be empathetic. We sympathize with each other about the future, and do not dwell on the fact that the "future" is much different for each of us.

It is as difficult for me to let go of my old ways of communicating, arguing, and getting what I want as it is for my caregivers. But for some reason, I keep expecting them to change by choice and by themselves, while I change because I have no choice.

Figuring out what is happening between my ears is of some comfort to me, but it scares my caregivers when I talk about it.

Hope and faith have been replaced with living today as if it were my last day of awareness, and reviewing the current abstracts of research focusing on how to slow down the disease's progress. I don't feel hopeless—I feel that to hope tomorrow will be better than today is a waste of time that diminishes my appreciation of today.

*Since I started writing, I am more confident and comfortable with who I believe I am.*

My spirit (whatever that is and means at any given moment) is shaken, weakened, and hesitant to express itself, but it is still alive within me. The harder I try to "be myself," the more problems I create for others. The more my caregivers cannot accept who I am, the more problems they create for themselves. They worry more about me. They must watch me more closely. My safety becomes more of an issue. The safety of others around me becomes more of an issue. They come closer to the day when they must decide they are no longer capable of keeping me safe.

I was not, am not, and never will be what others expect or fully want. I was mostly, am sort of now, and probably won't ever be what I expect or fully want. For me, losing control of myself—who I am, what I say, how I try to influence others to know me—continues to be very, very scary.

Since I started writing, I am more confident and comfortable with who I believe I am. I am marginally less afraid of the future. I have, I think, a better understanding of why and how I am changing; unfortunately, most of my insights come after the fact. I am mourning who I thought I was, and I am sometimes uncomfortable with who I am. The rest, I will just have to experience and hope I maintain some ability to understand myself from the inside out, as well as from the outside in, at least until I become engulfed by Alzheimer's rather than my current state in which Alzheimer's is becoming me.

# Dear Doctor . . .

To this day, many people are still confused between Ph.D. and M.D. degrees and between a psychologist and a psychiatrist. A Ph.D. is a degree granted by a college or a university to an individual who has completed additional course work beyond that of a master's level program and written a disseration. An M.D. is granted by a medical school for someone who has completed a course of study as a medical doctor. Psychologists are usually licensed by the state in which they practice therapy. They may not prescribe drugs that require a prescription. Psychiatrists are M.D.s who have completed additional training and study in the area of psychiatry and they can write prescriptions; they, too, are licensed by the state. Always ask if your physician, no matter what specialty she or he is practicing, is "Board Certified." This means he or she spent extra time as a resident, passed a pretty tough test in the area, and continues to keep up with knowedge in the specialty.

# If I Were an M. Instead of a Ph. D.

I would be aware that each patient's cognitive functioning is unique and that Alzheimer's presents itself as a syndrome (a group of symptoms).

I would be prepared to explain things to my patient as many times as it took for the patient to be able to explain it back to me in his or her own words.

I would never have more than three major points to make in any appointment with the patient. And, I would preview and summarize those points with the patient.

I would ask the patient to repeat the three points back to me in his or her own words.

I would never ask caregivers to speak with me outside of the hearing of my patient. If it was necessary for me to speak with them in private, I would call them.

I would always direct my remarks to the patient.

I would never act as if the patient were not in the room.

I would strive to help the patient feel as if this appointment was his or her appointment, not the appointment of the caregiver; as if the patient, lacking a sitter, was brought along.

I would understand that I probably will have to repeat what happened at the last meeting as a setup for what I want to talk about at this meeting.

I would never assume that the patient thought as I did. Nor would I attempt to convince the patient that he or she should.

I would take the responsibility to explain my thoughts in a manner which the patient understood.

I would be careful not to simply repeat myself.

I would schedule a double appointment time for the patient.

I would encourage caregivers to make their own separate appointments with me.

I would meet with a person with Alzheimer's in my office rather than in an examination room.

I would sit in a chair or on the couch next to the patient rather than behind my desk.

I would not wear a white coat when I met with a person with Alzheimer's.

I would always look the person in the eye when I was talking, and speak directly to him or her.

Early on, I would look for an opportunity to laugh with my patient.

Early on, I would talk about the past with my patient until we made a connection.

I would remind myself that my patient does not have dementia as a result of old age. He or she has Alzheimer's disease, which has its own unique, defined, and identifiable conditions.

I would familiarize myself with the unique conditions prior to meeting a patient with Alzheimer's. Walking in the door reading the chart does not reinforce a sense of connection.

I would *prescribe* caregivers and patients to become involved in their local Alzheimer's Association's groups and support services.

I would provide them with brochures that outline the Association's services.

I would follow up on my recommendations at the next appointment with the patient. I would write them down and we would all sign it.

I would ask my patient if he or she wanted to add any issues to my stated three goals/topics prior to beginning the examination.

I would ask my office manager/nurse to call the caregiver prior to an appointment and ask what issues he or she would like me to address.

I would look for opportunities to use psychopharmacology to help patients deal with the effects of the disease and medication.

I would realize that for the next few years, my role as a physician for the patient and family would expand.

I would call the patient the day after the appointment and speak directly to him or her and review what we had covered the day before.

A new case of dementia arises every seven seconds, reported an article in *The Lancet* (December 17, 2005). The report, produced for Alzheimer's Disease International, comes 100 years after the first description of Alzheimer's disease and estimates that 24.3 million people currently have dementia, with 4.6 million new cases annually. By 2040 the number will have risen to 81.1 million.

The study highlights that most people with dementia live in developing countries: 60% in 2001, rising to 71% by 2040. The rate of increase is predicted to be three to four times higher in developing regions than in developed areas. Already, many more people with dementia live in China and its neighbors (6 million) than live in either Western Europe (4.8 million) or North America (3.4 million). By 2040 there will be as many people with dementia in China alone as in the whole of the developed world put together.

There is already a great need for community-based services, welfare, and support for people with dementia and their carers. These new figures show that pressure on governments for dementia services will increase dramatically in the next few years, and governments must be prepared.

The report concluded that there needs to be a climate for change, but this must start by correcting a fundamental lack of awareness among policymakers, clinicians, and the public.

*http://www.alz.co.uk/media/nr051216.html*

# From My Heart to My M.D.'s Ears

Approximately four years ago, while driving my daughter, whom we hadn't seen in over a year, to the airport, she leaned over the back seat of our car and whispered in my wife's ear: "Something is wrong with Dad." Almost one year after, following dozens of tests, what seemed like quarts of blood, cups of spinal fluid, and hundreds and hundreds of repeated neuropsychological tests, my family and I heard the words: "You have dementia, probably of the Alzheimer's type."

After three more years of living with Dr. Alzheimer stomping around between my ears, leaving clumps of sticky plaques wherever he goes, I stand here charged with the task (by my own physician and friend, Dr. Victor Narcisse) of telling a group of noted internists and gerontologists "What's it like to have Alzheimer's disease?" And do it in less than eight minutes.

So—ready, set, go:

What's it like to have Alzheimer's disease? It's hearing my son tell me that I can't be alone with my five-year-old granddaughter because he is afraid one of us will wander off and forget the other one is there. It's having a family member, in a moment of frustration and anger, tell me that I am very selfish and have the emotional development of a 12-year-old because I want everything now. It's having my wife tell me wistfully sometimes, sadly sometimes, angrily other times, "You just aren't the same person I married." It's hearing a receptionist in a doctor's office who forgot my name say, "I guess I have a touch of Alzheimer's today." It's walking from the front yard to the back yard and not knowing why I am there. And repeating the same forgetful trip 10 or more times in an hour. It's listening to my friends talk and not understanding what the hell they are talking about because they are talking so fast and so many of them are talking that I can't follow the conversation. It's crying by myself in my own back yard and not knowing for sure why—just being sad in spite of Eli Lilly's and my doctor's best efforts to deal with my depression. It's hearing that one noted neurologist has recommended I need electroshock therapy, while another tells my wife in front of me that I need to come back to see him only after I have pulled down my pants and peed in the middle of my living room!

What living with the disease means to me, *really* means to me, is having to die twice in front of my family. First comes the death of who I am, and second is the death of who I will become. It means having to become an almost helpless observer of the deterioration of my relationships with loved ones. It means not remembering what I said, what I meant, and what you said or meant. I have moved from forgetful to confused to bewildered; I am floating between and within the three states, and I don't know why or how or when it is going to change.

I have moved from dozens of scraps of paper, each with an important "note to self" on it, to to-do lists, to multiple computer-generated to-do list alarms, to lists of to-do lists, to one day at a time, to simply caring less about what is and is not happening to me and my obligations to others.

What's it like to have Alzheimer's disease? What's it like to have ALS? What's it like to have a grand mal seizure, or a stroke, or to be blind? Difficult answer to fully appreciate for anyone who has not experienced it, because any illness affecting the brain affects in a unique way the way we perceive ourselves and our experience. I am fundamentally different from you. Different in ways I can't express and you can't fully perceive or understand. Our brains are different. You don't understand how your own brain works, and I don't understand how my brain works, and never the twain, at least for the foreseeable future, shall meet.

What's it like to have Alzheimer's disease? It's going to the doctor, lots of doctors. Most all of them seem to care, but unfortunately most all of them really don't know what to do about the disease or me. Please don't keep repeating to me what you think and believe, in hopes that eventually I will "get it." Don't talk louder in hopes I will "hear" you. Don't place your hand on my shoulder, bend over, look sympathetically into my eyes, and in lowered tones tell me what I obviously haven't and can't understand from your point of view.

People, including people in white coats, lose the extra credibility that my mom taught me when I was a youth to respect. I don't care if "the doctor told me to take my pills." If it's so important for someone to take them, then let him or her take them. I'm not interested in what the doctor thinks I should be eating or whether I should be driving or where they all think I should be going or what I should be doing. They are not me; I don't tell them what to do, so what gives them the right to tell me what to do?

What's it like to have Alzheimer's disease? I don't care like I used to care prior to my diagnosis. I still care if the referees make fair calls for the Chicago Bears. I still care about my family. I don't care about *me* in the ways I did previously. I don't want to die, but I don't necessarily want to live the way you think I should live, and I sure don't think God has suddenly decided that you or my family is smarter than I am about what is best for me. I don't believe that living without pain is necessarily the most important thing; it does not represent the quality of life I would prefer for the next few years while I sit in a wheelchair, mute and oblivious to my surroundings. I don't consider smiling at someone I know once or twice a week to be the level of human communication I want to enjoy for three or four years, while I fight off bed sores and have difficulty swallowing and trouble breathing.

And, by the way, please, please stop treating me like a child. You seem to have only two ways of treating me: either like an adult or like a child. I was and still am an adult. I don't feel like a child, and I am discovering that the only way for us to get along is for me to act like a child. I don't want to do this. Please don't help me become dependent on you and my family. Come up with some new ways to treat people with dementia that encourages, not discourages, them to be all they can be. Don't keep stressing what I can't do or shouldn't do. Figure out ways for me to do more, not less. Helping me is not just hindering me from doing things you believe I can't or shouldn't do.

> *What's it like to have Alzheimer's? Physicians assume they are in charge of me because of my diagnosis.*

Please understand, I live in a world with different paths than I used to walk, and certainly different paths than you walk or recommend to your other patients.

I'm not sure you have to eat every day to be healthy. I don't always believe I have to wash every day to be clean, and I'm not real sure about your clean hang-up anyway. And what's with this I "have" to take your medicine? Why? I don't always believe your advice is the best advice to help me.

What's it like to have Alzheimer's? Physicians assume they are in charge of me because of my diagnosis. I read on your web site that you take pride in practicing medicine derived from "Evidence-Based

Clinical Practice." We all know there is much evidence available on the diseases of dementia, but no one knows what it means to me as a patient. You all seem worked up over the fact you now have a drug to give me, which about 60% of the time helps people for three months to as long as two years. Well, what if I'm not in the 60%? What happens after three months or two years? Oh, it still may be having an effect, even if the quality of my life is deteriorating. Oh, I might be deteriorating faster if I wasn't taking the drug? Oh, and what about all these side effects from my depression drugs? Oh, and why suddenly can't I take drugs for my anxiety? Five years ago, I would have been peacefully full of them. Oh, and what about the fact that my level of acceptable risk for treating my disease seems to be increasing while you are waiting for evidence-based clinical practice guidelines. I told you we were different in ways neither of us can really appreciate in the other. Will you please work on this growing gap between us? Will you please bend, to create new models for relating to patients. I won't and can't.

How many of you have sat down for a couple of hours and talked with someone in the first and second stage of my disease? How many of you lived with someone like me for a week or two in medical school? How many of you really can claim you can answer the question: What's it like to have Alzheimer's? How many of you accept my claim that the diseases of dementia are different in fundamental ways from viral infections, from broken bones, etc. You don't have to break your arm to effectively treat it in someone else. You do have to spend more time with me, you do have to work harder with me, and you do have to become more involved with me and my caregivers to effectively treat me, because we are fundamentally different from many of your other patients. We are not just physician and patient; we are physician and individual living with one of the diseases of dementia. The differences seem to me to be very important to you, and I know they are to me. Please work longer, harder, closer, and differently with my caregivers and me, so we can all better understand what it is like to have Alzheimer's disease, and what each of us can do about the situation.

*We are not just physician and patient; we are physician and individual living with one of the diseases of dementia.*

What might it be like for you to have early-onset Alzheimer's and go into your office to see patients?

Arise at your usual time of a quarter to sometime. Shuffle into your kitchen to . . . can't remember. Shuffle back to bed. Arise at a quarter after in a panic because you are late. Start to shave and see your hairbrush and begin to comb your hair. Kiss your spouse or significant other goodbye and notice you still have shaving cream on half your face. Arrive at office and notice you are two hours late because you did not attend to the little hand on the clock, only the big hand. Also note that you didn't tie your tie. Slip into white coat and wonder why staff is staring at your feet. Meet first patient and bring in clipboard which vaguely resembles a chart but is in reality the list of lunch orders for the sandwich shop on the first floor. Start to ask questions and halfway through discover you haven't taken any notes, just asked questions. Your mind, which formerly produced questions that led to a diagnosis, now asks a lot of unrelated questions. The evaluation seems to be going nowhere. Reported symptoms, which previously would trigger specific questions, now are ignored. You comment on the faces of the people you saw as you drove in this morning. You interrupt the patient and ask why she is here. You move on to the next room and leave the first patient sitting. You assume the second patient is the first patient and begin diagnosis before the second patient begins to talk. When the nurse walks in, you ask who he is because you don't recognize him. As you sit down in your chair, you notice you still have your bedroom slippers on. Turn to patient and ask why he's here. Begin to cry for no apparent reason, and tell patient why you are so angry at your spouse for something you can't remember. Realizing how out of touch you are with what is going on around you, walk into waiting room and sit down and begin to read a magazine. Walk back into office and see the rest of your patients for the rest of the day and don't miss a beat. Forget most of what happened this morning but feel very embarrassed when you return home and your man or woman asks, "How did it go today, Dear?"

Each of these things, in one form or another, has happened to me, although not all in the same day and obviously not in a medical office setting.

I realize I wasn't invited here today to tell you what you are doing wrong, just what you are doing as seen through my eyes. I don't profess to lay claim to know what "the" Alzheimer's experience is or is not. I only know, sort of, what my experience has been. I am sure it's the same with each of you. None of you knows what "the" best physician–patient relationship is between a person with Alzheimer's and yourself. You only know of your own experiences, from your own perspective.

Please consider my words and what they represent. Please see if we can both get to trust each other more, to be aware, and to live under the assumption that each of us knows best a part of how I should be treated.

I want you to help me live as long and as healthy a life as I can. I want to help you to help me.

# Do No Harm

A year ago, I started to collect the occasionally obtuse answers physicians give to direct questions asked by patients who have been diagnosed with one of the diseases of dementia. This list includes contributions from me and from others, and let's be clear that they did not come from any of my current doctors. These are mostly word-for-word responses, although in the interest of amusing readers, I have exaggerated some of them. Know also they are not necessarily answers to the specific question, but they are answers given to patients living with one of the diseases of dementia. I don't claim that these are representative responses of all physicians. I collected them here to see if your physician has uttered one or more of them and to let you know that, if such is the case, you are not alone.

Me: Will this almost former hippie become aggressive?

Doctor: I can say with a great degree of confidence that the answer to your question is yes or no. We will have to wait and see what happens.

Me: Thanks! Will I be aware of my aggressiveness when it is occurring?

Doctor: That's a hard one to answer. You may or may not be aware of it, or you may be aware of it and not be able to do anything about it.

Me: Oh. I see! If I do become aggressive, what forms will it take, and what are the warning signs?

Doctor: (turning his head toward the caregiver who accompanied me and lowering his voice) Will he understand what I am saying? Does he bother you with questions like this, too? How long has he fixated on this issue? Now I know what you mean when you told me he can sometimes be difficult.

Me: Excuse me, doctor; I thought this was *my* appointment!

Doctor: Oh, so it is. Those are two good questions and I'm glad you asked them. I'm not sure how to answer them.

Me: Well?

Doctor: Do you have any more questions I can answer for you?

Me: Yes! Have any of your patients ever become aggressive with you?

Doctor: That was a problem for me, but I added those straps to the stirrups, and they really cut down on the aggressive behavior.

Me: No, I mean, have any of your patients with one of the diseases of dementia ever become so frustrated with you that they became aggressive?

Doctor: Usually not during my examinations, but sometimes during my Q and A with them they sometimes get worked up. I haven't figured that one out yet.

Me: Oh! Well, why haven't you answered any of my previous questions? What's the sense of asking more questions?

Doctor: Now hold on, here. Don't get aggressive with me. I've answered your questions as best I can. I encourage my patients to ask me any and as many questions as they want. I even encourage them to write them down before they come in to see me. I want to help put your mind to rest about things which are of concern to you and your caregivers.

Me: Oh?! Well, what have researchers discovered about patients like me and aggression?

Doctor: Has anyone ever told you that you ask extremely good questions?

Me: Yes, you did, about two minutes ago.

Doctor: Oh, I see. Well, again, you have asked an extremely good question. As best as I can tell, researchers fall pretty much evenly along the bell-shaped curved on this one. This is what a bell-shaped curve looks like. (Draws a bell with no ringer).

Me: Oh, I see. Would you recommend I change my medications or add a medication to anticipate aggression?

Doctor: You could, but then again, you might not want to. The decision, of course, is always yours to make. If I were you, I wouldn't quite know what to do. You have asked a very good and a very hard question to answer. Now, what else can I do for you?

Me: Oh? Well, would you please give me your best informed doctor's opinion? After all, that is why I came here.

Doctor: I was reading an article about that just the other day in a journal. (Pause while she/he looks for journal whose name she/he can't recall.) I can't seem to find it right now. Let me make a note on your chart, and the next time you come in I will be sure to have your answer.

Me: Oh! Do you review patient's charts before they come for their appointments?

Doctor: Of course I do. Any doctor worth her/his salt pauses outside the exam room door and thoroughly reviews the patient's chart before entering the room. We don't want to be embarrassed and forget your name or call you by the wrong name, you know.

Me: Oh? I see. Well, getting back to my original question . . . You know, I come here for answers I can't answer because I don't have your training and experience.

Doctor: Of course you don't. And I appreciate you choosing me as your doctor. You know, there are 34 other doctors just in this building alone. People don't always realize they have a choice, and it is informed consumers like you who keep us on our toes, so to speak. What other concerns can I help you with?

Me: Oh, well good for me and for you. What has been your experience with other patients in my position? What have they done? How did it turn out?

Doctor: I can't tell you their names. You know, patient confidentiality and all that damned government regulation. When I got out of medical school, people trusted and respected their doctors. They left their treatment in his/her hands, and we did what we thought was best for the patient. Now, do you understand why that's about all I can offer to answer your question and keep the FBI and the FDA out of my life and my office?

Me: I really don't need to know their names, just your experience treating them. Now what about aggression and me?

Doctor: That's a question I think is best answered by a psychologist. You need a couple of days of exhaustive testing, asking you hundred and hundreds of questions which will seem meaningless to you. After that, he/she will put them in a computer and the computer will tell us the answer to your questions. Of course, we will need the psychologist to sign the printout, so it is his/her report.

Me: I've already done that with different psychologists, and aside from the fact that one took twice as long to do it and charged half as much, they both reached the same conclusion—they couldn't say one way or the other, but they both thought it might or might not be a possibility depending on many factors, which they would try to identify if I could come back for a couple more days of testing. You are my M.D. What is your opinion?

Doctor:  Well, I'm glad you see it that way. Psychologists still can't make a medical diagnosis, and I hope that day never comes. But, really, I don't think I'm the best one to answer that question. That is a question you should, of course, ask a specialist. I understand you have an appointment with your (fill in the name of one of many specialists here—podiatrist, orthopedists who specialize in surgery for the smallest finger on your right hand, proctologist, ENT specializing in treatment [but not surgery] of the left ear hammer bone only, neurologist, etc.), and your appointment is only six months away. Why don't you write down your questions and ask her/him?

Me:  Oh. When should I come back and see you again?

Doctor:  Honestly, there is not much more I can do for you. Why don't you come back after you have pulled down your pants and peed in the middle of your living room? Then we can talk about other medications. (I admit, I am the one to whom a neurologist actually said this.)

Me:  Oh!?

Doctor:  Don't forget to stop by the front desk on your way out. It's how I stay in business, you know. I will have to code this as an established patient visit of extreme complexity and of unusually long length. Call me any time you have any more questions.

Me:  Oh! Thanks!

## THE COST OF ALZHEIMER'S CARE

- National direct and indirect annual costs of caring for individuals with Alzheimer's disease are at least $100 billion, according to estimates used by the Alzheimer's Association and the National Institute on Aging.

- The average lifetime cost of care for an individual with Alzheimer's is $174,000.

- Alzheimer's disease costs American businesses $61 billion a year, according to a report commissioned by the Alzheimer's Association. Of that figure, $24.6 billion covers Alzheimer's health care and $36.5 billion covers costs related to caregivers of individuals with Alzheimer's, including lost productivity, absenteeism, and worker replacement.

*http://www.alz.org/AboutAD/statistics.asp*

APPENDIX

# *What You Can Do*

# Taking Care of Your Favorite Organ

D on't be alarmed. This is not an unsolicited ad for Viagra from a pharmacy located in a rowboat floating off the coast of Kochi (formerly known as Cochin), a port on the west coast of India. (Doesn't the use of Mr. Google's tool add more interest and humor to writing, while at the same expanding our knowledge?)

For everyone over 50 years of age, a part of the yearly or biannual checkup should include a long-neglected organ, the brain! Call it *Remember Me, Don't Forget, Healthy Brain, Taking Care of Your Favorite Organ,* or whatever the universal program ends up titled, this action should establish for each of us a baseline of results against which we could measure the health of our brain, concerning issues of the diseases of dementia, every year or so.

Every year, we ask physicians to check out our hearts, our livers, our prostates and/or our breasts, and our eyes; but we almost universally neglect to check our brains. There should be a call to design a model that promotes and reinforces this primary care physician activity as part of a comprehensive plan to change how physicians and citizens understand and relate to the issues created by the diseases of dementia.

We haven't been able to scare folks with the certainty of the increase in the number of people with diseases of dementia—from 5 million to *15+ million* in the next 30 or so years—so perhaps we can convince them that it's in their own self-interest to take care of and monitor their own brains!

Individuals who are currently living with a diagnosis of one of the diseases of dementia are the best-informed, most-motivated, most-effective, and most IGNORED segment of the population to speak to these issues. It's time to work with US to enable us, not disable us; to speak to our needs and to your needs; to better understand, adapt to, and abolish the major stigma associated with growing old—forgetfulness. We need to respond to it for what it is: a group of diseases that can be treated (in some cases, and temporarily) but not yet cured.

Those of us with Alzheimer's disease do not become "stupid," or "dumb," or hard of hearing, or regress to childhood because of the disease. Yet, that is how we are treated. We can never be who we were and who many people still want us to be; we are who we are. We need others to become more informed, more understanding, and make more of an effort to understand us.

Dementia is a group of diseases and conditions that we do not yet fully understand. Therefore, unfortunately, we do not fully understand how and why they affect the people who are victims of these diseases. We banish people from our families because they don't fit in/take up too much of our time/disrupt the family, and we store them in small warehouses (nursing homes) until they die. We treat them like children because that is the only other way we know how to treat people, other than as adults. (We have pretty much given up trying to understand how to treat teenagers, but we know they will grow out of it, whatever "it" is.)

The best we can do, *right now,* is monitor ourselves for these diseases, hoping to identify and treat those who will be victimized by them. We must make more of an effort to understand those who have the diseases and listen to what they have to say, and to better support ongoing research to find the causes of and cures for the insidious diseases of dementia.

*Annual brain checkups are a good first step for everyone!* Please pass this idea on to three of your friends and ask them to pass it on to three more. Thanks.

# Best Friends

Currently there is a small evolution/revolution eking its way through the Alzheimer's community as to what is the most appropriate, least offensive, and best characterization of people who take care of someone who is living with a diagnosis of one of the diseases of dementia. Are they my caregivers, my caretakers, my carers, and/or my best friends? Which words best describe my relationship?

Is it really the words that make a difference or is it the philosophy? Currently most carers (that's the word used by the rest of the world other than the United States) have two general models of relating to other human beings: adult to child or adult to adult. I know teenagers are most often a class unto themselves, and what about those "I don't know or care much about anything" 20s, and the "what's in it for me" 30s, and so on. But basically we have two buckets of assumptions, practiced behaviors, and general ways in which we, right or wrong, treat each other.

When we discover we can't get what we want from individuals by relating to them as adults, we frequently shift to trying to get what we want from them by treating them like children. We tell rather than ask. We assume rather than explore. We talk rather than listen. We tolerate rather than accept. We sympathize rather than empathize.

This adult–child model, I believe, is what we adopt when relating to someone with Alzheimer's disease. It's more efficient and frequently more effective. There is another school of thought that says "tell them what they want to hear" (I call it *lying*), and another that says "distract them from what they want to talk about and bring them back to what you want to talk about" (I call it "pay no attention to their expressed needs"); focus on your own needs and what you know is best for them. Those two strategies could be the topic of an entire new book!

I want to encourage, advocate, promote, and persuade you to think about being a "Best Friend" to the loved one in your life who has Alzheimer's disease. I want you who are living with the disease to consider looking for more best friends in your life—not necessarily more children or spouses.

Think of what *best friends* means to you. How do you relate to them versus how you now relate to each other? I know he's your husband or she's your mom, but that old way of relating isn't working, is it? It makes everyone sad, mad, and frustrated that it doesn't work: the fact of the matter is, it doesn't work! End of analysis.

Two people, Virginia Bell and David Troxel, who have spent a lot of time with people like me who have dementia, developed the idea of reframing our relationships to one of best friends, regardless of what our real relationships are. They wrote a book about it, *The Best Friends Approach to Alzheimer's Care* (Health Professions Press, 2003, ISBN 978-1-878812-35-3), which I encourage you to please, please make your next book purchase.

From time to time, I bemoan the fact that I don't know how to relate to people now and they don't seem to know how to relate to me in a way that is best for me. Now I know! *Best Friends*. It's not the easy answer. The more deeply and longer you have loved each other, the more complicated it is. The longer you have each played a role other than that of best friend, the more difficult it is. Everyone talks about being a best friend; it usually starts in the wedding vows. Go back and check. It is time to act on that pledge. Read *Best Friends* and better understand how to practice what you began preaching years ago.

# Act Up! Act Out! Act Now!

To my companions on this road less traveled, the increasingly crowded Boulevard of the Diseases of Dementia:

While legislators (for whom we continue to vote and return to office) slip amendments into state and federal bills to make it harder and harder for children of the working poor to qualify for health care coverage, they turn their backs on us—their own grandmothers, mothers, fathers, cousins—and, in 10 to 20 years, themselves.

Diseases of dementia are real, and they are, for a large percentage of those growing old, inevitable. They strip our dignity, disrupt families, and contribute to other complications of our health that inevitably cause premature death. Every day, we know more and more about them. Every day, we realize how difficult it is to conquer them. As a large segment of our society moves into "the golden years," the possibility increases that a large segment of the population will deal with one or more of these diseases. As more of us reach our golden years, the diseases of dementia will seem to suddenly spread like an epidemic (although they are not contagious) through our families and friends.

It should be a crime against humanity for individuals with a confirmed diagnosis of some form of dementia to experience delays in receiving (and, in some cases, be denied outright) the benefits of disability insurance for which they have been paying the premiums for the past 30 to 60 years! I live in Texas, which has, to no one's surprise, one of the highest initial rejection rates for first-time disability claims in the United States. There are people living around me in this state who actually believe this is a good thing and are proud of our record. Shame, shame, shame!

Go figure—and people point to us and say *we* are acting irrationally? Why would we become hostile, paranoid, fearful, and depressed? After all, isn't there always a safety net to catch us if we are rich, raise peanuts, export military weapons, or build airliners for the middle class?

The fabric of American society is about to be stretched in many ways by the aging baby boomer population. There is already a large hole in the fabric through which many of us are falling or are destined to fall. After we have exhausted *all* our resources; after our Medicare benefits are once again readjusted because of the cash drain that wars have placed on our government; after we have lost our sense of self, our sense of dignity, we fall into a shaky and shrinking Medicaid system that no one wants to fund but everyone wants to keep as a "safety net" for their parents, and perhaps for themselves. We slip from one end of the long-term care facility with the fresh flowers and private rooms to the bare Medicaid wards in the distant wings of the facility. Now, legislators worry about funding the services for themselves and their peers. Not that they are doing a particularly good job at that, but where is the hue and cry for existing benefits that shrink every time a state legislature meets?

Evidently, these policymakers have each saved $400,000+ to cover the cost of 10 years in long-term care facilities for themselves, their parents, and the poor, whose life-long low wages made it impossible for them to save in the first place.

It's time for us to *act*. Research for AIDS did not achieve its present level of funding because everyone with AIDS stayed home and worked in their gardens. Friends of people with AIDS did not only worry about episodes of wandering and about keeping electrical outlets covered, they too *acted out*. They mobilized individuals with an interest in their cause and made acting as an advocate an expected part of dealing with the disease.

Think about this while you can. Act on it while you can. Act for yourself, your generation, and the future generations of your family and friends. Point out how you have been treated and/or ignored by the various systems in place that claim to exist because they want to support and help you. Write lots of letters. Send lots of e-mail. Speak in churches, schools, and council meetings. Don't stop until you have to, and trust that those after us will continue!

Caregivers who are filled with fear and depression, use this pent-up anxious energy to educate yourselves, your families, your friends, and those around you about how our society treats those with the diseases of dementia. If these organizations won't be worked up to action in the name of your loved ones, perhaps self-interest will motivate them. The bell tolls for us all; it is just a matter of time when and where we hear it. I've heard it. I have Alzheimer's disease.

**Act Up! Ring Out! SPEAK UP and OUT!**

# Web Resources

pproximately 60% of people diagnosed with one of the diseases of dementia probably have Alzheimer's disease. The rest of you probably, or maybe even for sure, have something else. It may or may not be reversible. It may or may not be treatable. Generally speaking, the other diseases of dementia, especially when compared with Alzheimer's disease, have been treated like orphan diseases by the public. For instance, Pick's disease has 1% as many hits on Google as does Alzheimer's. I am sorry I do not spend more time in the book or in these Web resources addressing the other diseases of dementia. Many organizations that claim to be focusing on dementia are in fact focusing on Alzheimer's disease. Great for me, bad for you. Write to me (richardtaylorphd@gmail.com) if you would like to do something to correct this injustice.

The Internet is never a substitute for human beings facing each other and supporting each other. However, it is not always possible for your supporters to be around when you want to talk, so chat rooms on a limited-use basis are okay—according to me. They are also a place to find people who live near you so you can get together and have a larger, face-to-face support network. I recommend three different chat rooms on Yahoo, because I read and participate in them on at least a weekly basis. I founded one, I am a moderator of one, and one I just enjoy. They are in Yahoo!Groups and they are: *Best-Friends-Alzheimers-Disease; alzheimers; and DementiaRescue.*

Google the names of all the drugs you have been prescribed. Check out each drug on WebMD, the drug manufacturer's site, and at least six other sites. You should end up knowing more about the drugs you are taking than the doctors who have prescribed them. The Web is the easy place to find that information.

Google the full name of every health care professional who is working for you. See what they have published. See what others have said about them in print. See what they have said about themselves.

Other than the book *Best Friends,* I have consciously not mentioned other books of, by, or for people living with the disease and/or their caregivers. Most of them have something of use, but you must decide what. Go to a book store; find all the books by people who have

Alzheimer's and/or their caregivers and page through them. When you find a couple that seem to be of value to you, buy them. Or, go to your local library.

No printed list of Web resources can ever be up to date or comprehensive. Ask Mr./Ms. Google for Alzheimer's information and you will be led to more than 62,000,000 sites. Which ones are current? Which ones are best? Sorry, but you will have to decide that for yourself. Here are some sites I have visited since my diagnosis.

## Alzheimer's Association
### http://www.alz.org

The Alzheimer's Association is a national voluntary health organization supporting Alzheimer's research and care. On this site, you will find lots of information about Alzheimer's disease, programs, services, and advocacy. Start with this site, and pay special attention to their toll-free 24/7 help line. It is simply the best! Link to the local chapter nearest to you. The call to your local chapter should be your first call after hearing the diagnosis. They have "been there and done that," and they want to help.

## AARP
### http://www.aarp.org/

AARP is a nonprofit membership organization dedicated to addressing the needs and interests of people age 50 and older. Through information and education, advocacy, and service, AARP seeks to enhance quality of life by promoting independence, dignity, and purpose. They speak with one strong, loud, and *listened to* voice concerning issues of seniors.

## Alzheimer's Foundation of America (AFA)
### http://www.alzfdn.org

AFA is a national organization dedicated to supporting individuals and families dealing with Alzheimer's disease; it is an excellent "first" source to consult. Subscribe to their free caregivers magazine. Contact their partner organizations. Quality service, in a timely manner, is provided by people who obviously care. Phone: 866-AFA-8484.

## The National Family Caregivers Association (NFCA)
### http://www.nfcacares.org/

NFCA is a caregiver membership organization that provides services in the areas of information and education, support, public awareness, and advocacy for caregivers. Phone: 800-896-3650.

## National Respite Locator Service
http://www.respitelocator.org/index.htm
This organization helps parents, caregivers, and professionals find respite services in their state and local areas. Call your local chapter of the Alzheimer's Association first, and then call these folks: 800-773-5433.

## Leeza's Place
http://www.leezasplace.org/
It was Leeza Gibbons's dream when the Foundation began that it would offer a safe setting for all families who are dealing with loved ones diagnosed with a memory disorder. This site, Leeza's Place, is a community-based oasis for caregivers and the newly diagnosed that practices what it preaches. It is a "must visit."

## Family Caregiver Alliance
http://www.caregiver.org
The Family Caregiver Alliance is a nonprofit organization that addresses the needs of families and friends providing long-term care at home. It has developed a wide array of services based on consumer needs and is often described as a "one-stop" shop for caregivers.

## Alzheimer Forum
http://www.alzforum.org
A compendium of information for researchers, physicians, and the general public, the site includes news, articles, discussion forums, interviews, diagnostic and treatment guides, and directories of drugs, clinical trials, and research advances. It also provides access to unique tools such as directories of genetic mutations, antibodies, patents, and conferences.

## Alzheimer's Disease Education and Referral Center (ADEAR)
http://www.alzheimers.org
ADEAR maintains information on Alzheimer's disease research, diagnosis, treatment, drugs, and clinical trials. Find out if there is an ADEAR center near you. It is a source of consistently superior care, information, and referrals.

## Medline Plus: Alzheimer's Disease
http://www.nlm.nih.gov/medlineplus/alzheimersdisease.html
An all-in-one search site, this page provides links to recent news items, symptoms and diagnosis, research, statistics, clinical trials, coping issues, and other resources.

## Federal Citizen Information Center
http://www.pueblo.gsa.gov/cic_text/health/alzheim/brain.gif
The image illustrates degenerative neurons in the brain and the areas responsible for motor, vision, sensory, speech, and memory functions.

## Alzheimer's Disease Process (film clip)
http://www.nia.nih.gov/Alzheimers/AlzheimersInformation/GeneralInfo/
In an 80-second film clip, learn about neurons, neurotransmitters, tangles and plaques, and the death of nerve cells.

## Normal and Alzheimer brain comparison
http://www.alzbrain.org/quicklinks/picturegallery.htm
See lateral and overhead scans of a normal brain and an Alzheimer brain, with labeled areas of memory, understanding, hearing, speech, temper, personality, and brain atrophy.

## Mayo Clinic Alzheimer's Disease Center
http://www.mayoclinic.com/health/alzheimers/AZ99999
The Mayo Clinic site contains articles on driving, caregiving tips, nutrition, communication, stress management, depression, interactive caregiver stress tools, and a free e-mail update service.

## Planning for Long-Term Care
http://www.niapublications.org/agepages/longterm.asp
This web site from the National Institute on Aging explores the options for long-term care, with articles on planning ahead, making the right choice, and making a smooth transition.

## Predicting Time in the Nursing Home
http://cpmcnet.columbia.edu/dept/sergievsky/predictor.html
Columbia University has developed a tool to help predict how long it might be until a person with Alzheimer's requires nursing home care. See the home page for their methodology.

## Rush Manual for Caregivers from Rush Alzheimer's Disease Center
http://www.rush.edu/Rush_Document/CaregiversManual.pdf
Written for family caregivers, the manual contains chapters on stages, treatment, communication, intimacy, coping, spiritual needs, legal

matters, traveling, driving, exercise, hygiene, incontinence, nutrition, and more.

### Washington University in St. Louis: The Alzheimer's Page
http://www.biostat.wustl.edu/alzheimer
This site links aging and dementia sites and contains the Alzheimer discussion group (an on-line support group for family caregivers and professionals).

### Alzheimer Disease International (ADI)
http://www.alz.co.uk
The ADI web site links to more than 77 Alzheimer's disease associations throughout the world, primarily in developing countries. It lists information about AD (for the person with AD and the caregiver) in English and in more than 25 languages. It also contains information on the global impact of Alzheimer's as well as on activities of ADI.

### CNN Health Library: Alzheimer's Disease
http://www.cnn.com/HEALTH/library/alzheimers/
CNN's site has basic information about Alzheimer's, as well as topics such as communication, sleep problems, end-of-life needs, and more.

### Alzheimer's: Information for Kids and Teens
http://www.alz.org/Resources/kidsandteens/overview.asp
This page provides resources to help kids and teenagers learn about Alzheimer's disease and understand how it affects them.

### Helping Children Understand Alzheimer's
http://www.cnn.com/health/library/HQ/00216.html
CNN/Mayo Clinic offer help with questions that children may ask about Alzheimer's.

### ClinicalTrials.gov
http://clinicaltrials.gov
People with Alzheimer's disease, family members, and members of the public can find current trials and research. The searchable database provides information on the name of the study, the purpose, eligibility, and contact information. In addition, the site indicates whether the study is recruiting and includes citations from published works.

## AARP: Life Answers
http://www.aarp.org/life/
Life Answers is a series of on-line articles sponsored by AARP. Topics include caregiving, driving safety, legal solutions, grief and loss, independence, and housing.

## Brain Teasers
http://www.hlavolamy.szm.sk/brainteasers
A variety of brainteasers and logic games

## Brain anatomy SPECT images
http://brighamrad.harvard.edu/education/online/BrainSPECT/Contents.html
Brain images of different types of dementia

## Alzheimer's, Dementia, & Driving
http://www.thehartford.com/alzheimers/index.html
This site, developed by the Hartford Insurance Company, helps families cope with the dilemma of persuading a family member with Alzheimer's to stop driving. I am not keen on recommending information provided by commercial organizations, but this is excellent information, and the problem is universal for families dealing with Alzheimer's disease.

## American Medical Association (AMA)
http://www.ama-assn.org/ama/pub/category/5099.html
On-line resources from the AMA about the health consequences of caregiving.

http://www.ama-assn.org/ama/pub/category/5037.html
A caregiver self-assessment tool developed by the AMA to monitor caregiver stress levels.

## Ageless Design
http://agelessdesign.com
Sign up today for their free daily update on news and views (yes, I write a monthly column for them) in the Alzheimer's community.

## Alzheimer's: Understanding Changes
http://www.alzheimersdisease.com/info/answers/understanding-changes.jsp?checked=y
Explains changes that occur with Alzheimer's. This is a site from Novartis (a pharmaceutical company), so be forewarned.

## American Health Assistance Foundation
http://www.ahaf.org/alzdis/about/adabout.htm
Offers health care assistance to those in need.

## Dealing with Dementia
http://www.ncpamd.com/dementia.htm
Ways of dealing with dementia

## Neurology Channel
http://www.neurologychannel.com/dementia/diagnosis.shtml
This site explains different types of dementia and seizures.

## Northwestern Research Center for Alzheimer's Disease
http://www.brain.northwestern.edu/
Northwestern Research Center offers information about various forms of dementia.

## Popcap Games
http://www.popcap.com/
Find a variety of fun games to play and relax with.

## Because We Care: A Guide for People Who Care
http://www.aoa.gov/prof/aoaprog/caregiver/carefam/taking_care_of_others/wecare/wecare.asp
The Administration on Aging has an on-line resource guide for the growing number of Americans who are caring for an older family member, adult child with disabilities, or older friend. This guide provides information and a range of suggestions to make caregiving easier and more successful.

## A Year to Remember: Alzheimer's Book Reviews
http://www.zarcrom.com/users/yeartorem/bkreviews.html
Here are some reviews of books about Alzheimer's and caregiving.

### Caregiving.com
http://caregiving.com/landing.cfm?loc=index.cfm
This site contains on-line articles on caregiver issues. It includes stages in caregiving, a caregiver support center, frequently asked questions, and caregiver stories.

### National Association of Professional Geriatric Care Managers
http://www.caremanager.org/
This site describes the role of the care manager and allows users to search for a local certified geriatric care manager.

### National Council on Aging: Consumer Information Network
http://www.ncoa.org/content.cfm?sectionID=209#cin
NCOA provides short education programs on topics such as Medicare, Alzheimer's, safety, relationships, and other issues of interest to seniors.

### National Institutes of Health (NIH)
http://www.nih.gov
NIH offers information about clinical trials and information about dementia.

### Nursing Home Info
http://www.nursinghomeinfo.com/
Nursing Home Info provides information about choosing a nursing home, listings of facilities, and a needs assessment tool.

### AgeNet Solutions for Better Aging
http://agenet.com/
AgeNet Solutions for Better Aging provides articles on caregiving, housing, legal matters, insurance, health, home, and drugs. It also provides on-line tools such as an eldercare and a home safety checklist.

### American Geriatric Society (AGS) Foundation for Health in Aging
http://www.healthinaging.org/
AGS Foundation for Health in Aging provides consumer-oriented research from the American Geriatric Society. A complete on-line book, called *Eldercare at Home,* focuses on the health problems of seniors.

### U.S. Department of Health and Human Services: Eldercare
http://www.eldercare.gov/
The Eldercare Locator allows users to search for eldercare resources in any state.

### Eldercare Advocates
http://www.eldercareadvocates.com/
The Eldercare Resource Center provides a variety of articles on all aspects of caregiving.

### ElderWeb
http://www.elderweb.com/
This is an excellent site for news updates on legislative, health, legal, and consumer protection issues.

### U.S. Administration on Aging
http://www.aoa.dhhs.gov/
Official Web site of the Administration on Aging. This U.S. government site describes programs and services for seniors which are funded by the Older Americans Act.

### FirstGov for Seniors
http://www.firstgov.gov/Topics/Seniors.shtml
FirstGov for Seniors is a user-friendly site that compiles health, consumer protection, and legislative information from other government sites. Much of the information is health focused.

### Medicare
http://www.medicare.gov/
This is the official U.S. Government site for people with Medicare. It has information about Medicare benefits, nursing home comparisons, Medigap insurance, prescription drug assistance, and more.

### Center for Medicare Advocacy
http://www.medicareadvocacy.org/
The Center for Medicare Advocacy helps seniors and people with disabilities understand Medicare benefits and obtain needed services. Extensive information on Medicare rights can be found here.

## GovBenefits
http://www.govbenefits.gov/
GovBenefits provides brief information about social security programs, with on-line forms and applications.

## Connecticut Partnership for Long-Term Care
http://www.opm.state.ct.us/pdpd4/ltc/home.htm
CT Partnership for Long-Term Care provides information about purchasing long-term care insurance. The site lists plans and describes how the Partnership can provide long-term care insurance savings.

## National Senior Citizens Law Center
http://www.nsclc.org/
The National Senior Citizens Law Center advocates nationwide to promote the independence and well-being of low-income older individuals and people with disabilities.

## Social Security Online
www.ssa.gov
Social Security Online provides information on all social security programs.

## Connecticut Legal Services, Inc.
http://www.ctelderlaw.org/
The site is sponsored by Connecticut Legal Services, Inc. and offers articles on nursing homes, patient rights, wills, funeral arrangements, health care, and where to get legal help. Extensive information is provided about Medicare and Medicaid. Want to or not, you are going to become an expert on Medicare and Medicaid. This is a good resource.

## National Academy of Elder Law Attorneys, Inc.
http://www.naela.com/
NAELA's consumer section contains articles on how to select an elder law attorney. The site allows users to search for the names of elder law attorneys in all states. Yes, they can be expensive, but they know what they are doing and we need their knowledge!

### Eldercare Online Legal and Financial Channel
http://www.ec-online.net/legalchannel.htm
Eldercare Online Legal and Financial Channel provides articles on elderlaw, financial matters, taxes, estate planning, and more.

### NoLo Law for All
http://www.nolo.com/
NoLo's Retirement and Eldercare section provides articles on financial matters, estate planning, advance directives, and so forth.

### Aging with Dignity: 5 Wishes
www.agingwithdignity.org
The *5 Wishes* document helps you express how you want to be treated if you are unable to speak in your time of need. *5 Wishes* also encourages discussing your wishes with your family. It is the most sensitive, comprehensive, and clear living will I have ever seen. I have it. You should, too! Go visit this site and have everyone in your family complete one for him- or herself.

### AARP Legal Solutions
http://www.aarp.org/families/legal_issues/
AARP Legal Solutions provides articles on legal matters and practical tools such as a worksheet for your will.

### American Bar Association Consumer's Guide
http://www.abanet.org/public.html
The American Bar Association consumer's guide to help on the Internet provides articles on working with lawyers.

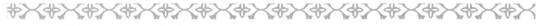

## *A NOTE FROM MY GRANDMOTHER*

When I was a young boy, my already-aged grandmother would raise a quarter-filled glass of Mogen David wine at Christmas and remark that it was so wonderful that the entire family was able to get together because this was probably her last Christmas. She died when I was 47!

Merry Christmas everyone!

*Richard*